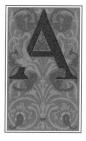

Almond Eyes
Lotus Feet

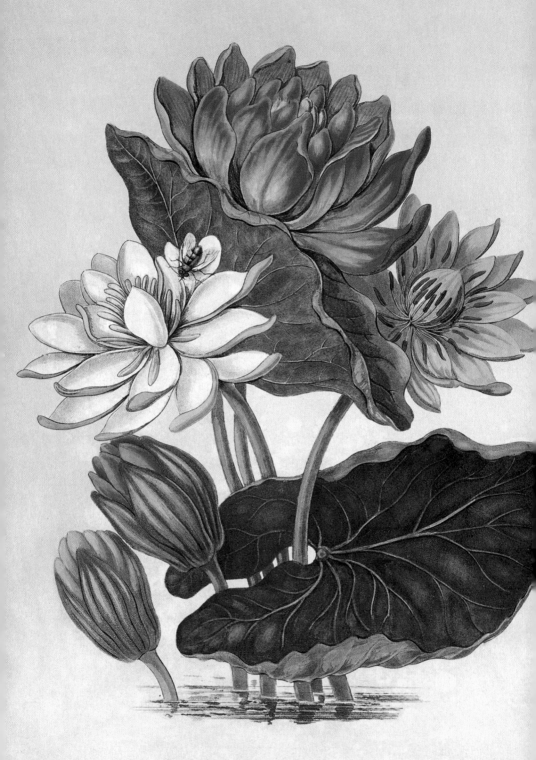

Red, Blue, and White LOTUS, *of Hindostan.*

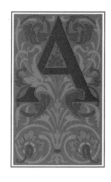

Almond Eyes
Lotus Feet

INDIAN TRADITIONS IN BEAUTY AND HEALTH

SHARADA DWIVEDI • SHALINI DEVI HOLKAR

With a foreword by
Princess Esra Jah

Collins

An Imprint of HarperCollins*Publishers*
www.harpercollins.com

Originally published in India by Eminence Designs Pvt. Ltd in 2005.

ALMOND EYES, LOTUS FEET. Copyright © 2007 by Sharada Dwivedi, Shalini Devi Holkar. All rights reserved. Printed in the United States of America. No part of this book may be used or reproduced in any manner whatsoever without written permission except in the case of brief quotations embodied in critical articles and reviews. For information, address HarperCollins Publishers, 10 East 53rd Street, New York, NY 10022.

HarperCollins books may be purchased for educational, business, or sales promotional use. For information please write: Special Markets Department, HarperCollins Publishers, 10 East 53rd Street, New York, NY 10022.

For editorial inquiries, please contact HarperCollins Publishers, 10 East 53rd Street, New York, NY 10022.

FIRST EDITION

Designed by Dhun Suresh Cordo

Library of Congress Cataloging-in-Publication Data has been applied for.

ISBN: 978-0-06-124653-1
ISBN 10: 0-06-124653-0

07 08 09 10 11 * RRD 10 9 8 7 6 5 4 3 2 1

For our daughters, Sabrina Holkar and Radhika Dwivedi, with much love.

Contents

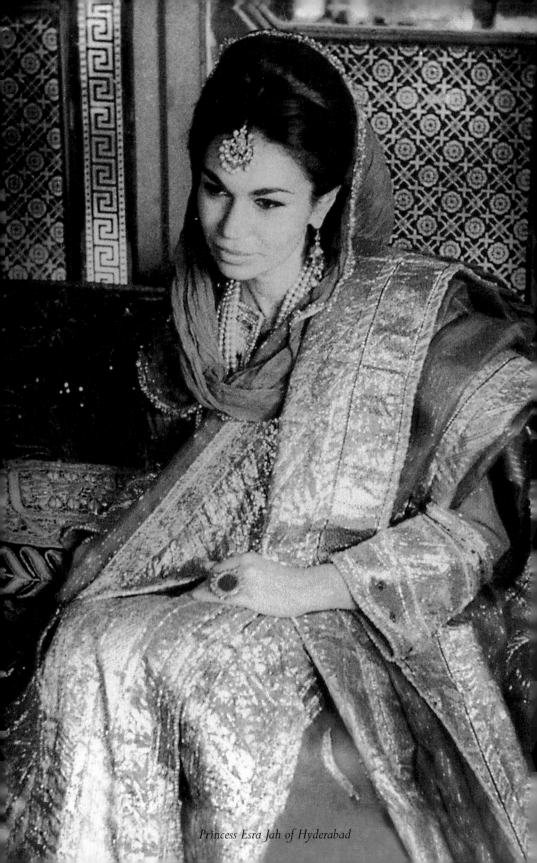

Princess Esra Jah of Hyderabad

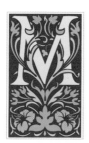

Moments of Grace

Whenever I read an article written by people settled in other countries using flowery language I am a little suspicious of its sincerity. However, at risk of making the same mistake myself, I must say that I find most Indian women not only extremely beautiful but also appearing to possess great inner strength and wisdom.

For me, outside beauty must reflect what is inside and I have seen these qualities over and over again in many women during my time in India. They have taught me their patience and how to treat difficult moments in one's life as tests to be overcome. After twenty-five years away from India coming back was like returning home, my friendships as strong, warm, and supportive as if I had never left.

I find Indian women have great physical advantage. They are usually born with lovely eyes and teeth, beautiful hair and skin. I remember spending hours with my hair in coconut oil and my body in pastes made from special ingredients, trying to achieve the luxurious hair and smooth skin of those surrounding me.

In those days, it was fashionable in Europe to sunbathe for hours to get a tan, yet Indian women were trying to whiten their skin . Now, years later, they have come to realize how intrinsically beautiful they are, enabling them to win beauty competitions all over the world!

The graceful movements are seemingly inbred in all Indian women. To walk down a village road and see them carrying their wood piles or pots on their head is to realize the inborn grace they possess. They are courageous enough to wear the most brilliant colors, and on them it appears luxurious:

all the colors provided by nature are displayed in their garments. Even the simplest sari looks elegant.

I have always loved the sari. When I was a young girl an Indian friend of my mother's was visiting us in Istanbul and I asked permission to see her saris. When she saw me looking at them with such joy she said, "Well you must marry an Indian so that you can wear them." Little did she know that this would become true. When I married into the Hyderabad family my chance came to wear the sari and I loved it. In the beginning I wore them with difficulty but with the help of my friends I finally learned the art.

When Nizam VII died and my husband succeeded, one of my first visits was to the storerooms where the old materials and saris were kept. I felt as if I were in Aladdin's cave: there were rolls of textiles, old costumes, and cupboards full of saris. But as I touched them, I found to my sorrow that most of them crumbled in my fingers due to years of not being aired. Luckily we managed to salvage at least some of them.

The more I look into the adornment of women the more I see the importance of taste in the use of jewelry. From ordinary silver anklets to the most lush jewelry in India there seems to be sophisticated taste, however humble or grand the wearer may be. The uncut form of stone used in Indian jewelry has a magnificence that cut stones do not possess. Indians seem to have an ability to mix colors, both in jewelry and in textiles, in ways that are exquisitely harmonized.

How strange it is to reflect that the young generation in India is now trying to copy Western dress, whereas Western fashion is looking toward ancient Indian inspiration for glamor.

Esra Jah

PRINCESS ESRA JAH
LONDON, 2005

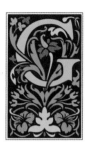arlands

They are all Padmini, all the women who shared with us their own ideas and expertise, the fruits of a long life of experience. As we have gathered from each of them to give to Padmini, so Padmini must give thanks to them.

Many have now left us, but we have fond memories of them all. To each of those wonderful people we offer a fragrant garland of gratitude: Qamar Ahmad, Ameneh Ahmed, Farida Ahmed, Baiji, Rajmata Pravin Kunverba, Princess Shri Kumari of Banswara, Durga Bhagvat, Princess Padma Lokur of Bhor, Minnie Boatawala, Vandana Chatterjee, Dr. Sharadini Dahanukar, Princess Shashiprabha Raje of Dhar, Maharani Brijraj Kumari of Dhrangadhara, Princess Sitaraje Ghatge, Lady Fay Holkar, Mayadevi Jain, Janaki Joshi, Sushila Joshi, Sati Kaul, Anjanabai Lolekar, Hansa Mariwala, Habiba Miranda, Leela Moolgaokar, Shanti Moti Chandra, Mayarani Mukherjee, Savitribai Nene, Indumati Phadke, Begum Maqbul Jehan of Palanpur, Maharani Perveen of Pratapgarh, Prema Ramakrishnan, Nirmala Sharma, Sonibai Shinde, Princess Vijayraj Kumari of Udaipur, Princess Rukmini Varma of Travancore, and Maharani Rama Kumari of Wankaner.

And to the men who helped us in many ways, a scented bouquet with many thanks: Dr. Ravindra Bapat, Appashaeb and Subhash Pethe, Sulaiman K. Shama, Brigadier K. C. Sharma, and Cory Wallia.

We are grateful to Rani Nirmala Raje Bhonsale of Baroda-Akalkot, Harsha Dehejia, Princess Shashiraje Wallia of Dewas Jr., Radhika Dwivedi, B. D. Garga, Hemlata Jain, Sangita Sinh Kathiwada, Jimmy Ollia, Geoffrey Roome, Azmat Syed, K. V. Talcherkar, and Princess Rukmini Verma of Travancore who were so generous with illustrations and offer them our heartfelt thanks.

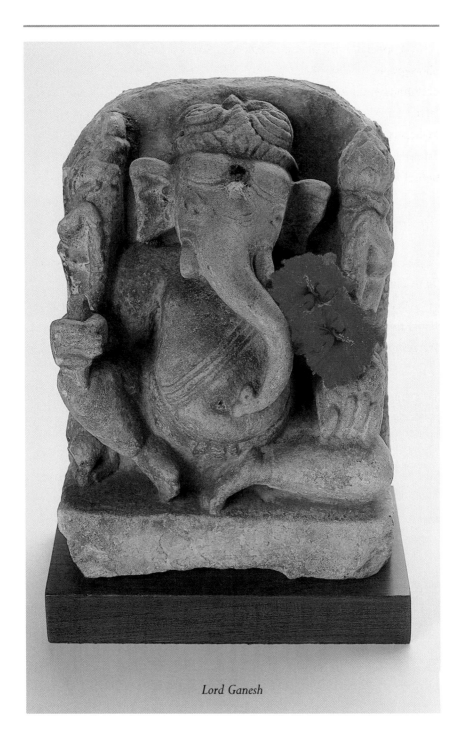

Lord Ganesh

A special word of appreciation to Suresh Cordo for his exceptional photographs of artifacts and Noshir Gobhai of the ingredients, to Farooq Issa of Phillips Antiques, who has always been so generous in sharing his vast collection of lithographs, postcards, photographs and company drawings and to Maharaja Ranjitsingh Gaekwad of Baroda, managing trustee of the Fatehsingh Museum Trust for permitting us to use images from their collection of Raja Ravi Varma paintings.

We offer a lovely lotus to Anna Bliss and Cassie Jones of HarperCollins and a fragrant magnolia to Marc Gerald of The Agency Group who fortuitously discovered the book during a trip to India. We are grateful to Eminence Designs, who originally published the book in India.

Princess Esra Jah of Hyderabad, a true symbol of grace and beauty, very kindly agreed to write a personal and enchanting foreword to the book. We are grateful and offer her a special garland of fragrant wild roses!

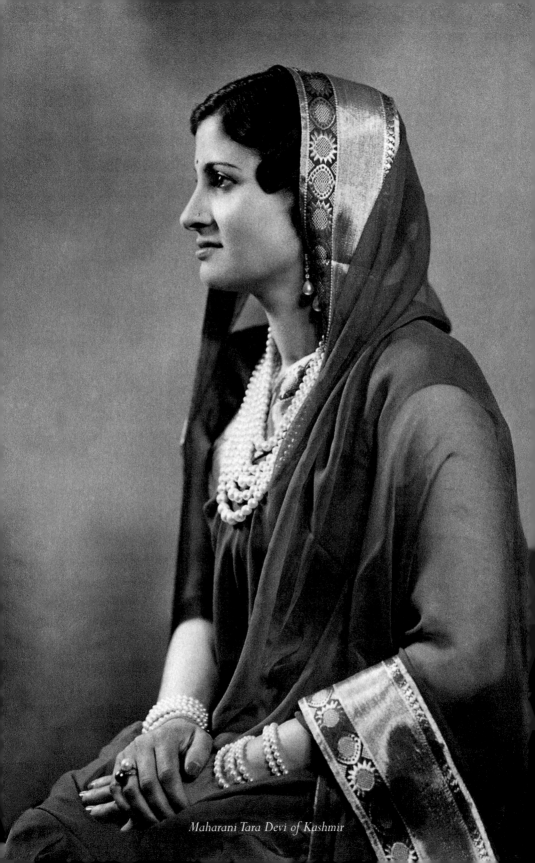

Maharani Tara Devi of Kashmir

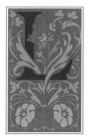oving Human Hands

"Granny, I love you dearly, but this book is a mess!" That's what my granddaughter said. I know what she meant: it is a hodgepodge—part first aid, part folklore, and part cookbook. I suppose in some places it's a bit naughty too—I mean, I talk about sex and such things. But the way we were taught, they're all interrelated. All the beauty secrets, the home remedies, and all the rituals I know at the age of seventy-five come from the same source: other women. I suppose that women practice these things for the same reasons: to keep everyone healthy and happy.

My granddaughter thinks I'm old-fashioned. I don't care. I shall put this all down as a labor of love, because there was so much love in it all. I guess that's what I see sitting here in Bombay today, looking back over the years. Indian women of my vintage were naïve, we were chattels and mere childbearers, if you like. Certainly we were not liberated, not even very well educated by my granddaughter's standards today. Almost everything we knew, we learned from our mothers and grandmothers and from other women around us. Maybe much of it was old wives' tales. Most of it certainly centered on one goal: grow up chaste, get married fast, produce a family, maintain a household, and never dishonor your husband or his family.

Beauty care was part of this ultimate goal and part of maintaining a delicate balance in life. Performing elaborate beauty rituals and using home remedies at least gave us the feeling that we had some defense against harsh climate, health problems, and wagging tongues in the family—all of which could unbalance life badly. Of course, there was the question of vanity too, but we never really thought of beauty care as a matter of fashion. We thought of it as tradition, obligation, habit, health care, and yes, as good recreation. It was such a lot of fun! Women were always together for massaging, bathing, washing hair, and even tending children.

My granddaughter finds the whole thing appalling! A big bunch of ladies in women's quarters—no privacy! No mind of your own! Everyone braided and beaded the same! Same spot on the forehead, same hair parting, same toe rings and bangles, same saris! I can see what she means, but we all felt very comfortable doing those things. They were rituals. We were all enacting the ideal wife myth we had read and heard so much about. The ideal wife in India has nothing to do with fashion. She is pure, modest, self-effacing, and literally worships her husband. In our days it meant that she covered her head whenever he entered her presence and she never ever uttered his name because the evil eye might fall on it.

Our evil eye obsession! Miss Blake, my governess, used to laugh. But God knows that eye could take away our children, husbands, health, and happiness if we dropped our guard even for a moment. Maybe that's why we all rushed to get married, have children, and get them married. Then we could see their children and be reassured that our line would continue. Seventy-five is not so very old, but I remember when women had no other recourse, no defense against the evil eye except our traditions, our so-called old wives' tales and home remedies, and by that I mean beauty care, too. Beauty care and hygiene were one and the same, both for ourselves and for our children as well.

I may have grown up in one palace and spent my life in another, but I know the evil eye made no exceptions. Rich and poor, we feared it alike and that fear made us respect things my dear Miss Blake never knew of or chose not to notice, things like the demands of the seasons. The unbearable heat and dryness of summer, the damp of monsoons, the all too brief chill of winter—each dictated a different regime. Then there was the matter of the qualities in articles of everyday use: were the spices "heating" or "cooling," was that beauty mark auspicious or inauspicious, were the metals in that food bowl beneficial to the body or not?

We had to consider all of these aspects even for a small matter like making lampblack for our eyes or for buying a stone from the jewelers, and certainly for big matters like marriage-making. Miss Blake never really understood such considerations and neither do women of my granddaughter's age—perhaps because they have lost touch with the earth. In Madanpur the earth was part of our lives; the gardens, grasses, flowers, and trees were like friends whom we trusted to help.

My granddaughter has always lived in a city. When she married she moved into her own home. Her children were born in hospitals. Her hair is bobbed and her nails are painted. She works, wears pants, and was schooled in England. She cannot imagine how life was for me before Granddaddy died and I left Madanpur to come to my Bombay apartment.

In some ways, she reminds me of my own, dear English Miss Blake, my instructress in so-called civilized ways. Miss Blake came to me in Madanpur after my marriage to teach me King's English and proper English manners. I was fifteen at the time. It took her a long time to accept our ways, just as my granddaughter finds them strange now. Miss Blake was horrified by many things when she first came; I was the child-bride she'd read so much about.

In the beginning she used to sit in the palace, in the women's quarters where we all stayed, and lecture me about matters like knives, forks, and spoons or the ungraceful act of staring. But she herself stared, because there we all were, oiling our hair, rubbing ourselves with strange concoctions, or just giggling about men—I am sorry to say—most irreverently for chaste young women. She must have thought we were awful. I can see all that now; our mouths stained with betel, bodies jingly with jewelry, big hips and bare feet, red with henna.

There she was fresh from England. We thought she was funny! How we stared at her: short hair like a widow, freckles on her arms (we were great ones for unblemished skin), a man's type of watch, and two little pearl earrings. We thought her very strange, almost an object of pity, were it not for her blue eyes and pale complexion, both of which we envied madly.

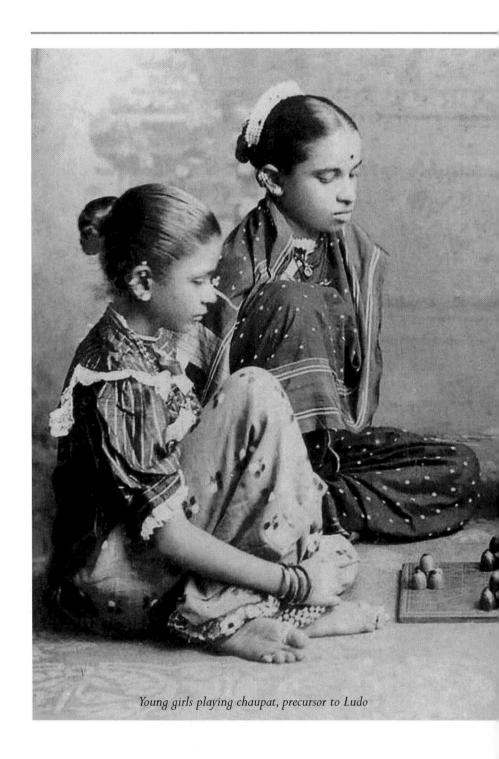

Young girls playing chaupat, precursor to Ludo

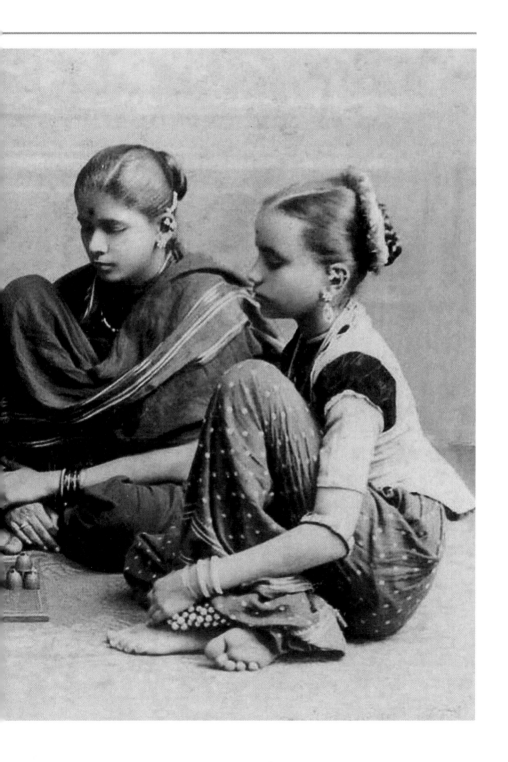

And she was supposed to teach *me*! As it happened we taught each other over the years. I grew very fond of Miss Blake. What I know of the world, I learned from her. And what she knew of India, I suppose we women all taught her, the ladies of the Madanpur palace. As my friends, tormentors, and accomplices, the palace women taught me "this mess," as my grand-daughter would say, this storehouse of knowledge I shall now record for posterity.

First I must make one thing clear. I know this seemed strange to Miss Blake. When I was a girl and a young mother, even though I was a princess, I used the same beauty secrets that my maids did, though perhaps I spent more time on them.

I had no bottles or jars or nice tubes of ready-made cosmetics. Everything we used, from creams to contraceptives, came either from the garden, kitchen, or herbal doctor. I can't tell you how different that was from what I see today, and how much more comforting. Modern women seem to have no clue, but we knew exactly what we were using or giving to our children to take.

We brushed our teeth with a twig from the big neem tree in the court-yard, cleaned our faces with earth from the river, and washed our hair with shampoos from the kitchen like yogurt and coconut water. As far as I know, women all over India were doing more or less the same thing. They had no choice beyond the garden, grocer, and old herbal doctor. But in India, nothing is true everywhere. Some women use one thing, others another. We are so many and so diverse, so I certainly cannot speak for all Indian women. But life has been good to me.

I have seen a great deal not only in Madanpur but also during travels with my husband after marriage and through social work here in Bombay. I have had a chance to compare the way different women behave, the way they beautify or bejewel themselves, and the rituals they perform for themselves and their families. So many of them were incomprehensible—even ridicu-lous—in the eyes of my beloved Miss Blake, but I know that many of them were basic and sound commonsense principles. They worked and kept us healthy and happy.

I will describe them and offer them to you with some of the images and memorabilia I have collected over the years—prints, postcards, and advertisements, photographs of old friends, and the work of our own court photographer who often traveled around the country with his camera.

I do not know if the treatments and recipes I have collected over the years from family members and friends always work. But they are intriguing and oftentimes romantic—and many are time-tested. Of course, everyone has to be careful of allergies to certain products, even natural ones.

As the saying goes, I do not presume to explain all, but perhaps I can enlighten. "Knowledge is in the heart, not in books." So I shall put my heart in this book.

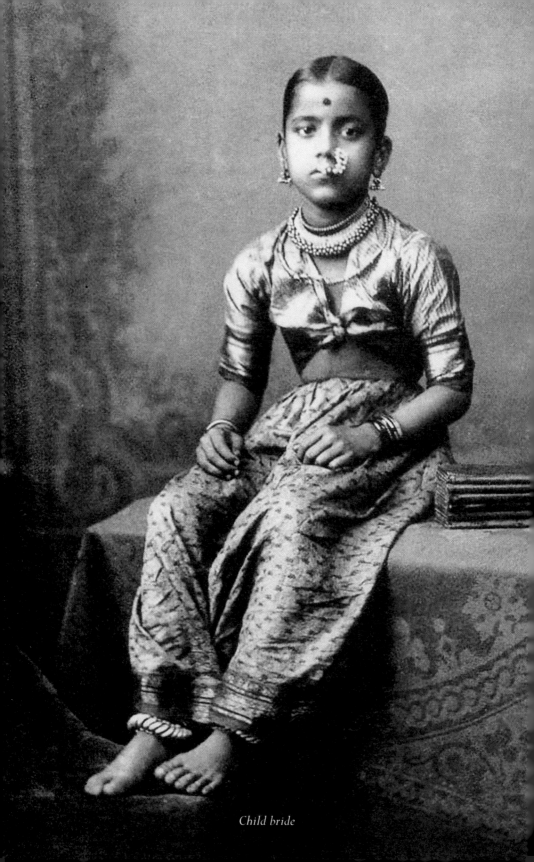

Child bride

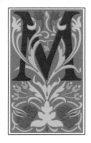arriage Mantra

I was born in Rajasthan in a small princely state. My father was its ruler, the Maharaja, and so I was a royal princess. When my five brothers were born before me, there was great rejoicing and beating of gongs. But when I was born, there was silence.

Rajasthan lies in the west Indian desert. It is a land of forbidding forts and great chivalry, but it does not welcome the birth of a girl any more than the rest of this land. I have heard that in Rajasthan, many newborn daughters were put in earthen pots and buried in the sands. That was before my time, but those were my people nonetheless: warrior caste Rajputs, sons of kings, sons of the sun and moon, according to legend. We are a race that takes the greatest pride in upholding honor.

I grew up hearing tales of Rajput women committing *sati* to avoid dishonor, burning themselves on their husband's pyres to fulfill dictates of honor. That part did not appeal to me although we were supposed to esteem such dedication to husbands. I did question *sati*, but somehow I never questioned my status as a female, a creature of quiet submission. Everyone I knew took it for granted that women were under some male's protection: their fathers and brothers until their marriage, their husbands after marriage, and their sons in their old age. It was understood that those men might do as they liked—short of fleeing from a battle—without incurring dishonor.

A Rajput's ideal woman was Padmini. Padmini was a legendary princess of Rajasthan whose husband was captured in battle when she was still a young woman. Rather than submit to the desire of the conquering king, Padmini threw herself into the fire. She was brave and she was also exceedingly lovely. So my father, with great hope, named me Padmini.

Poor father! I didn't live up to his expectations, I'm afraid. I was never very brave nor the least bit beautiful, but my mother always said that didn't matter. A woman's beauty, she said, was not just in her face, but also in her demeanor, in the goodness of her thoughts and her heart. My name means "lovely lotus flower."

There was talk of my marriage from the time I was a child. "A daughter and a bullock are always in bondage" is one of our proverbs. Another says, "Daughters: their coming makes you weep and so does their going." No one rejoices when females are born, but how everyone wails when the wedding is over and the bride departs with her husband to take up her new, married life. According to our customs, once a daughter is married, she no longer belongs to her father's household. She is gone! She belongs to her husband and to his parents, and she must honor and obey them forever. A common saying is "An unmarried daughter in the house is like an elephant." Marriage is not an option with us; it is an obligation. In their old age poor parents do not want another adult mouth to feed, nor do any parents want the shame of a spinster daughter, for it means they have failed in their duties to her. Sons on the other hand are very useful. They earn, support their elderly parents, and, when the time comes, perform their parents' death rites—something a daughter cannot do, according to our customs and traditions.

Daughters are expected to leave. So for many reasons the status of married women—we call them *suhagan*—is much coveted. That is why we Hindu women very proudly wear our *tilak*, the spot on our foreheads, which shows that our husbands are still living. Even unmarried young girls wear the *tilak* spots because we believe that though she may not yet be married, every young woman's future husband has already been born and awaits her somewhere. At all cost women must show the world that they are not widows! They wear their bangles and their *mangalsutra* necklaces (our form of wedding rings) proudly and conspicuously. Even if her marriage is unhappy, she wears them, because the worst fate that can befall a woman is widowhood. As a widow so many things are forbidden. Not just the *tilak* or *tikka*, the *mangalsutra* and the bangles, but also the wearing of colored clothes, the eating of spicy foods, and, in the olden days the company of others. "A woman without a husband is like a field without an owner." Long ago it was considered unlucky to look upon a widow's face because doing so could spoil your whole day!

So my granddaughter says I did well to come away from Madanpur and the palace when Grandfather died. Bombay is a much freer place. I do not think of myself as a widow living here. I even wear a small *tikka*, though I haven't the right, because the memory of my husband is with me still and he would have wanted it thus—just as he wanted me to give up *purdah* when we married.

Purdah is something Miss Blake never approved of, though I think she may have come to enjoy it. *Purdah* means curtain. Indian women lived as though behind a curtain, sheltered from the eyes of the world. *Purdah* was not originally an Indian tradition. It came several centuries ago with the Muslim invasion of this country. Muslims kept their women in a *zenana*—a women's quarter. Miss Blake used to call it a harem. Technically our faces, not to mention our bodies, were not to be seen by any but our husbands. In our day, the rules were not so strictly enforced, but there was a time in Indian history when the rules were so extreme that a woman would boast that "not even the eye of the sun had ever seen her sheltered face." In Madanpur we never took things that far! We kept our heads covered with the ends of our *saris* or long scarves called *odhnas* or *dupattas* that we wore with long skirts and tight-fitting blouses.

We were certainly modest in the presence of our elders or any of the men in our house, and only went out in cars with elaborate curtains and rail carriages with tinted windows. Whenever we went from the palace to the car, we were screened by a small mobile tent! It seems absurd now, sitting here in Bombay and moving, as I do, quite freely. But I know women of my age who long for *purdah* and miss covering their heads and faces like they did when we were royal *zenana* ladies.

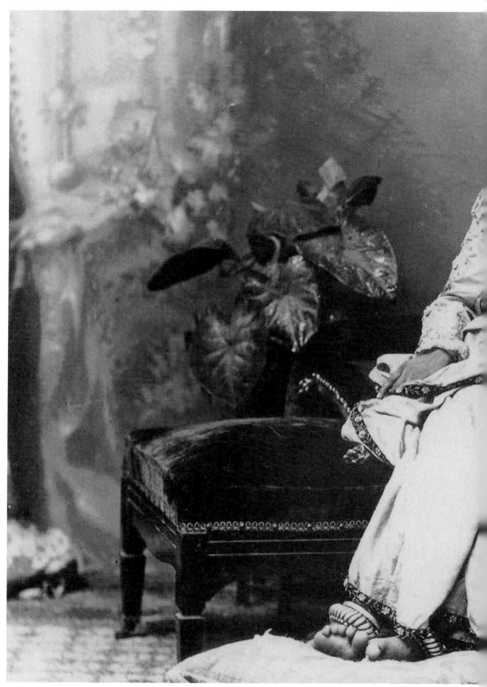

Young bride from Hyderabad

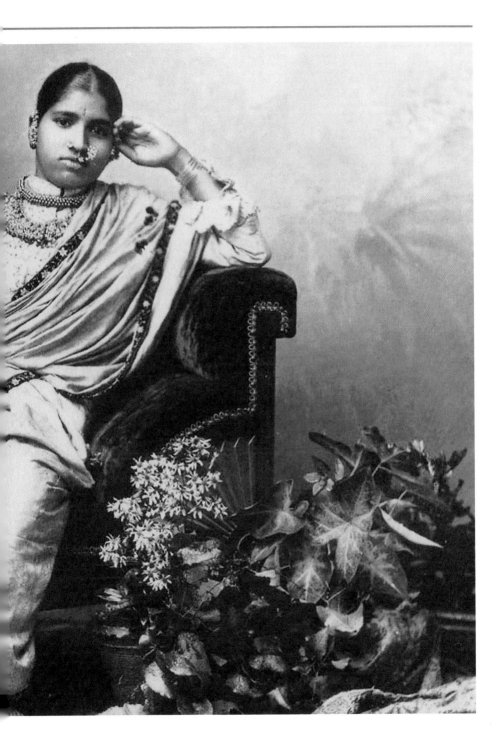

I've made a point of all this because then it is clear why we made so much fuss over our brides and why a girl's whole youth was devoted to learning how to be an excellent wife. As young girls we had little time for formal education; we were taught as much as the women around us knew. I was lucky—I had Miss Blake to teach me because both my father and father-in-law agreed that I should be educated. Most women learned only by example. Village girls learned their mother's tasks very quickly: sweeping, cooking, caring for the smaller children, and observing the many religious rituals, however elaborate or simple.

Palace women, however, knew little of such things. Work was left to our servants and maids. We very rarely did physical work or any form of exercise, first because it was considered beneath our dignity, and second because of *purdah*. Our education had much more to do with etiquette and demeanor. We learned respect for our elders, modest speech and action, and perfect execution of all the *pujas* or religious rituals. These seemed to fill up the whole year.

We also had to learn the *sola sringar*, the sixteen arts of beauty and adornment that every accomplished woman should know. I can't remember them all now, but they included bathing with various earths and unguents, anointing oneself with different oils, braiding the hair in a variety of styles, and rubbing scented essence into the body. We were also taught the art of adorning oneself and one's garments with jewels, how to wear caste marks correctly, and the appropriate dress for every season and occasion. Further, we learned to decorate our hands and feet with henna designs, to weave various types of flower garlands, and even the art of preparing and eating *paan*. *Paan* is the betel leaf into which we package spices and pastes and pop into our mouths throughout the day, like other cultures smoke cigarettes or take snuff.

We were taught all these things, but we were never taught about matters like menstruation! I find that hard to imagine now, because I grew up surrounded by women. I was engaged to be married at the ripe age of six, but nobody thought to tell me so much as one fact of life, not even my maids or my beloved aunties! They also betrayed me in this respect although I had always thought we shared everything like sisters.

Now that I have met so many other women throughout the country and have had a chance to talk to them, I realize I was not alone in my ignorance in thinking, when my first periods came, that I was suffering from some sort of shameful disease. I'm sure village girls knew much more about the birds and the bees than palace women did, though my maids still protest that they don't know much.

In any case, it was a favorite aunt who enlightened me when at last I gathered enough courage to tell her that I had been bleeding for three days and was surely dying. After she had reassured me and explained everything, I finally understood so many incidents which until then had totally mystified me.

ou see, Hindus consider a menstruating woman to be unclean. She must remove herself to a special room for three days and can have no physical contact with anyone, because her very touch would be polluting. According to our traditions, she cannot bathe for those three days and she must eat out of separate dishes. There is no question of her going into the *puja* room or kitchen. To this day, people will swear that a menstruating woman can spoil certain foods and make them unfit for eating, just by touching them with her hand!

As soon as my aunt explained about menstruation, then the whole thing began to make sense. Finally I understood the mystery of those poor women huddled into that small room. The maids forbade me to go there, telling me all those women had to sit apart from us because they'd been polluted by the touch of a crow. Imagine!

The crow is always the culprit in India! People blame crows for all sorts of things. When I was a little girl, I listened to the story but I refused to accept it. Once I went into the forbidden room in defiance of everybody. I hugged my favorite aunt who was sitting there and, to my great shock, she pushed me away. Before I knew what had happened, she'd stripped off my clothes and sent me off with the maid for a bath.

I wept with humiliation but never understood her action until my time came to sit in that room. You sat for three days and on the fourth, had a bath, washed your hair and performed a little ritual *puja*. After that you could do anything you liked. It was the same for every Hindu woman, whether princess or a peasant. The custom is still followed in many rural areas. The whole thing became a little less offensive to me when I realized that those three days of isolation were probably precious to hard-working women as the only respite they ever got from their unending succession of household tasks.

Still, I have a grudge against crows!

In the wisdom of old age, I have come to understand—if not to accept—the rationale behind so-called child marriage. Our society sets much store by virginity. Parents were naturally anxious to see that they delivered their daughter intact to her groom, so the sooner, the better, they felt. And perhaps they were right. The code of ethics was so strict that a bride could be rejected, a new marriage broken, if there were any reason at all to question that bride's virginity.

Muslims are particularly strict in these matters. In some parts of India, members of the groom's family actually stand outside the bedroom door on the wedding night, waiting to be shown a fresh stain on a white handkerchief, which is kept under the bride's pillow especially for that purpose. If it is not stained, God help the bride's family. That is ground for instant annulment and the girl will have no second chance!

Once they reach puberty, daughters are forbidden any activity that might possibly endanger their so-called key to that coveted marital status. Horseback riding, cycling, tree climbing—all of those joys of childhood are finished. Because of *purdah*, I could never do any of those wonderful things except in the presence of my brothers. But how I missed them after that wretched crow came to sit upon my shoulder and sent me off with the other women.

My father settled my marriage when I was six; but the wedding took place when I was fifteen. My father and my husband's father were friends and

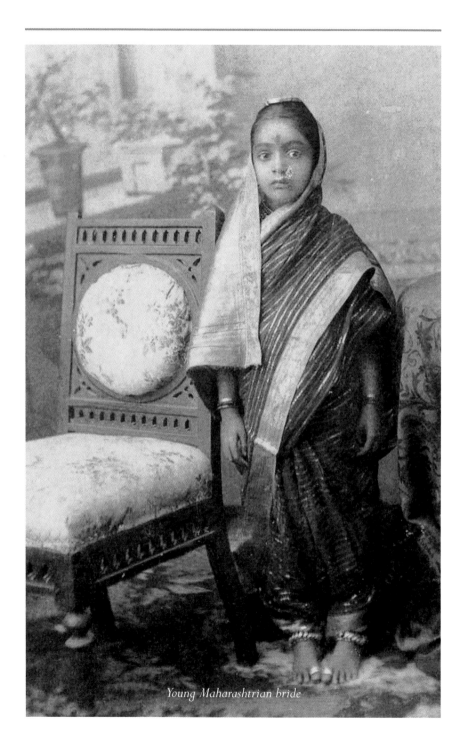

Young Maharashtrian bride

fellow students at the Mayo Princes' College. They agreed that their children should marry because our horoscopes matched very beautifully according to the *Raj Vaid* or court astrologer, who was also the ayurvedic physician. Madanpur is a much bigger and very much wealthier state than my father's little principality, but my clan of Sisodias is considered superior to that of my husband. For us Rajputs, caste and clan are very important. So the match met with everyone's approval as an appropriate alliance.

The nine years between my engagement and my marriage were spent learning to be a woman, especially to be a wife and daughter-in-law. An unseen husband is the object of one's dreams during those years, but an unknown mother-in-law is a dreaded nightmare. The thought of her strikes terror in many a young girl's heart. Will she be strict? Disapproving? Impossible? A terrible taskmaster? A good grandmother? Often a new bride's marital bliss depends not so much on her husband himself as on her relations with his family and particularly with his mother.

After all, they live together, and mother-in-law rules the roost. Next in importance comes the eldest brother's wife and so on down the hierarchy. When a new bride comes into the house, there seems to be some sort of unspoken agreement, especially among the women, that she must prove herself in every respect. She is unworthy until she proves otherwise and sometimes members of the family are merciless in testing her.

So she must conduct herself very wisely, maintaining good relations with all the relatives, obeying her parents-in-law's wishes, pleasing her husband in thought, word, and deed, and conceiving as soon as possible. Conceiving was very important and meant a son, not a daughter. Meanwhile there were many duties and responsibilities.

Palace women did not have to work, but we did have to learn how to run a household. The key word in all matters was *saleekha*. *Saleekha* is an Urdu word from the courtly language of the Mughals; it means balance and moderation, neither too much nor too little, but just the right amount in everything. Be it spices in the curry or smiles in court, they had best not be in excess or wanting. The other Urdu word drilled into our heads was *tameez*, which is respect and courtesy. There never seemed to be enough of that. We spoke in the politest form of our language, addressing people always in the formal *aap* form, never in the familiar *tum*. "You" or *tum* could be construed as too familiar or in some ways insulting, so even to servants we always spoke very politely and formally. *Tameez* involved elaborate procedures of etiquette, especially the touching of feet, a sign of respect in our culture. Women in most parts of India must bend from the waist and touch the feet of their elders when they meet them, particularly their parents-in-law.

I saw a lot of feet during my wedding ceremonies! My own became quite familiar to me because a bride is not supposed to lift up her eyes. She is meant to be a bundle of blushing modesty. I was exceptionally shy, and also sad at the thought of leaving my family and going away to an unknown place with a man I had never even seen. So when the time came during the ceremonies to lift my head and look at him, I simply couldn't open my eyes.

 must tell you that those eyes were elaborately prepared for this wedding business, as was every other square inch of me! For three weeks before the wedding ceremonies began, I was submitted to every traditional treatment ever known to the women of my "harem."

There were unending fragrant massages! My maids made up unguents known as *peethis*, a kind of cream made of oil, ground almonds, turmeric powder, a pinch of saffron, and a few drops of rose or sandalwood essence to enhance the fragrance. Turmeric powder is believed to be extremely auspicious, antiseptic, and cleansing. Turmeric and saffron are both used to impart an attractive olive glow and sheen to dark skins. They do impart a glow, but they stain clothes terribly!

For those massages I wore stain-proof yellow clothes and seated myself in the *dagla*, a cloth canopy specially constructed on the terrace of the palace. It was an elaborate ritual. Five women stood in attendance, one holding a ceremonial sword, while seven ladies of our Sisodia clan crossed their forearms, dipped their hands in the *peethi* concoction, and began to rub it on my body. They rubbed it into my feet, hands, cheeks, and head; always in this

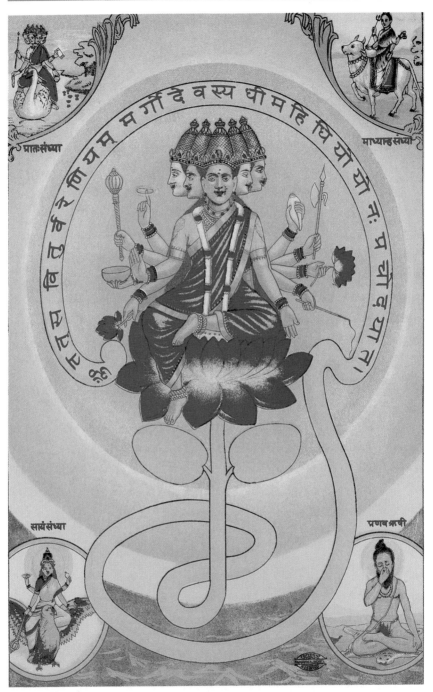

Gayatri Mantra

order, from bottom to top. This went on for seven days, then on the day before the wedding the order was reversed and the *peethi* was rubbed downwards from the head. Needless to say, there was a lot of singing and music during the *peethi* and the women teased the life out of me, but I was not allowed to protest.

Bridal preparations similar to this take place in many parts of India. The unguents used depend on the region. The idea I believe, was to render the bride as soft-skinned, clean, and sweet smelling as possible. It is true that at the end of it I was very highly polished and my body was literally permeated with a fragrance that lasted for weeks. I have heard that occasionally this sort of massage is done not by the bride's people, but by the women of the groom's family. Their mission is sometimes more than just a pleasant massage. They keep their eyes open for any blemishes on the bride's body, like a big mole or a scar, that might not have been mentioned during discussions for the marriage contract. Such blemishes are considered serious drawbacks and the groom's family might have to reconsider the match if the women bring home very bad tidings!

I was oblivious to all this during my massages, half in heaven at the thought of my forthcoming marriage, half in misery at the unending fuss!

Besides the *peethi*, there is another ritual, which is an absolute must for a Rajasthani bride and for many brides in India; it's known as *mehndi*. Miss Blake called it henna. Without *mehndi* there could be no wedding—that's how highly it is regarded. *Mehndi* is a squishy green-brown paste made from the leaf of a scrub bush, which grows in everyone's garden. For some reason, the goats will not eat it, so it is quite commonly used as hedging. We use *mehndi* paste to stain designs on our hands and to give sheen to our hair and our skin.

There is a saying that a person with unseen qualities is like a henna leaf, with its hidden color. Although the henna leaf is green, its stain leaves the skin red. When the leaf is ground with water and mixed with lemon juice and sugar, it makes a dark, pungent paste with an earthy aroma. We

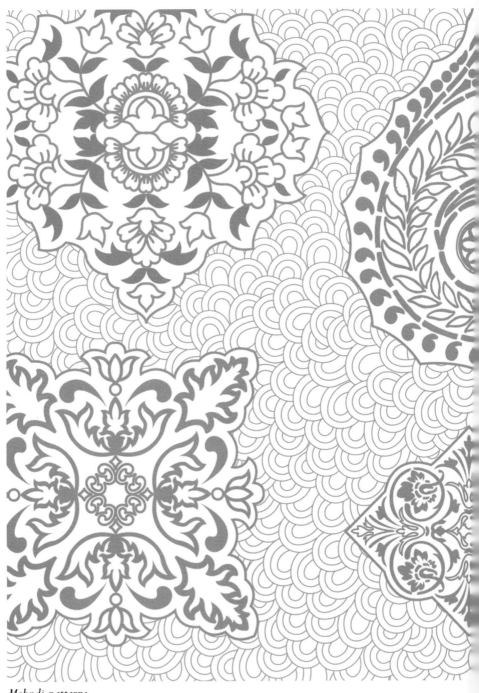

Mehndi patterns

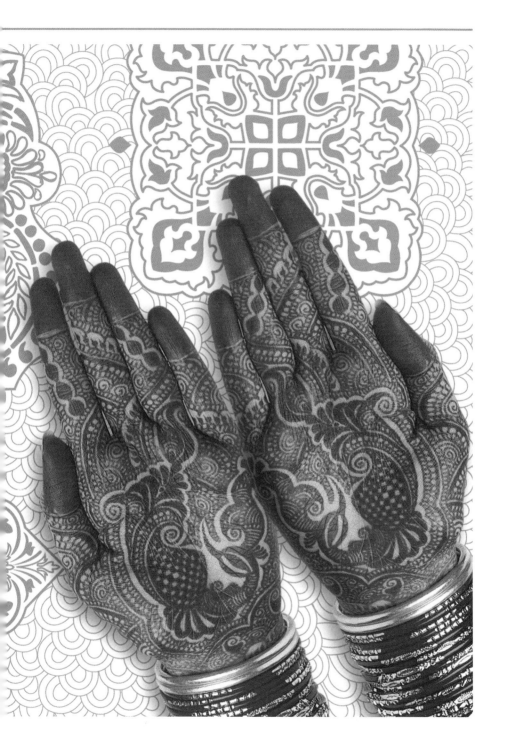

apply it on our hands and feet in intricate patterns and those patterns turn a deep reddish orange on the skin. If the paste is well made, the stains remain several days. We consider this an indispensable and a very auspicious ritual for every bride.

ll the women attending the wedding will also put on *mehndi* and it will be sent on a tray to each honored guest as a sort of gracious way of saying, "Come, join the fun, adorn yourself with auspicious *mehndi* like the bride herself is adorned." *Mehndi* is symbolic of the wedding in several respects. For example, only brides can wear *mehndi* on their hands and feet. Unmarried girls cannot wear it on their feet, and widows cannot wear it at all. There is also an additional meaning, a secret shared by the bride and groom on the wedding night and spelled out in the *mehndi* design. In Rajasthan, the bride's left hand is intricately patterned with intertwined flowers and leaves by women expert in this art. Artfully hidden among this pattern of foliage and leaves is the name of her future husband. The right hand remains unadorned.

That is the most exciting part, because a bride knows that her very first physical contact with her husband will be when her right hand clasps his right hand during the ceremonies. His right hand will have wet *mehndi* paste in it as well as a solid gold coin. I can still remember that first timid touch, holding his hand and hoping the *mehndi* would stain very dark.

It did, you know, and we had a good marriage just as the old beliefs promised. We also had a lovely time on our wedding night finding his name in the foliage. There is something to be said for tradition. Over the generations our elders have devised a number of such sweet games to break the ice and help overcome the awkwardness of newlyweds on their first night together. Palace girls were unbelievably innocent, for having grown up surrounded by women. I'm sure village girls knew much more than we, having lived much closer to their mothers and fathers and much closer to Mother Nature. We knew nothing. So we played ice-breaking games under the eyes of our elders and in this way, for some girls at least, the whole business of staying for the first time with your husband became easier.

Girls who were engaged and actually married before they reached puberty didn't go to live in their husbands' homes until they had their first monthly periods. Those first periods were occasions for great celebration. The girl in question was much pampered by the elders of the family.

There were endless wedding rituals and celebrations. For example, the bride and her husband were seated in a flower-decked arbor where they played games like "share the betel." Each one took a bite of a betel leaf *paan* (the spice-filled leaf that Miss Blake never liked) and laughed over who could get the bigger portion, without touching the other's lips. Then they made up rhymes with each other's names. The girl would be very coy, as she really didn't dare pronounce her husband's name for all to hear. There was always the evil eye to consider!

My husband and I passed much of our first night together laughing like the children that we were. He found his name among the *mehndi* foliage in my hand; then he spent hours undoing my hair. I've always suspected the maids had that in mind when they did my hair in such intricate braids intertwined with ever so many flowers the afternoon of the wedding.

It was my turn after that. I had to undo all the tiny little knots his sisters had tied in the drawstring of his silken *pyjamas*. Sweet frustration. We couldn't stop laughing. But I know I was lucky. What stories I have heard over the years from women who were much less lucky than I, mere children encountering their husbands on that first night without the slightest inkling of what to expect. It's quite amazing for a country which is known everywhere as the land of the Kama Sutra. Have we always been so inhibited, I wonder? Or is it a legacy perhaps from Queen Victoria when we were a part of the Raj?

I returned to my own home on the morning after my marriage. My sister-in-law met me at the door and put *mehndi* on my feet to signify that I was really a married woman. When I left home, I remember my mother's parting words, "Never disobey your new family, my darling. A Rajput woman does not think of herself, she thinks only of her family's welfare."

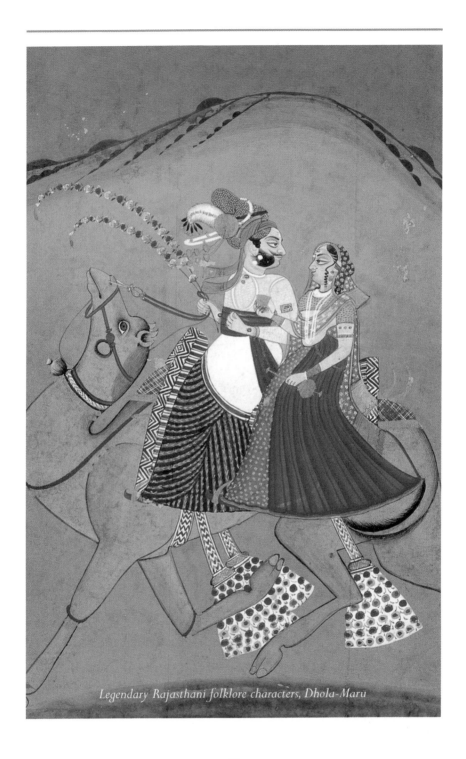

Legendary Rajasthani folklore characters, Dhola-Maru

ood thing my granddaughter wasn't there to hear that! But I never questioned my mother's advice and I never regretted that either. I did regret leaving my home, at least for a little while. All my sweet, silly, much beloved women, the bane of Miss Blake's existence, gathered to sing traditional farewell songs:

"Oh my love," says the bride, "turn your camel around, I miss my father,"

"Your father-in-law will fill the void in your heart, my fair beloved,"

"Turn back your camel my dearest."

She implores, "I want to bid good-bye to my mother once more!"

"Don't pine for her my doe-eyed one, your mother-in-law will love you dearly."

And so on they sang. I guess they're quite sentimental, all of these songs, but they're so much a part of our lives. We sing them so often that they become our dear friends, just like *mehndi* and all the other beauty secrets and elaborate rituals that my mother taught me so long ago and I still use to this day.

Miss Blake found the rituals messy and unesthetic. I can still hear her using that word. But she and her husband Major McBride must have missed something on their honeymoon night with no names to look for in the foliage!

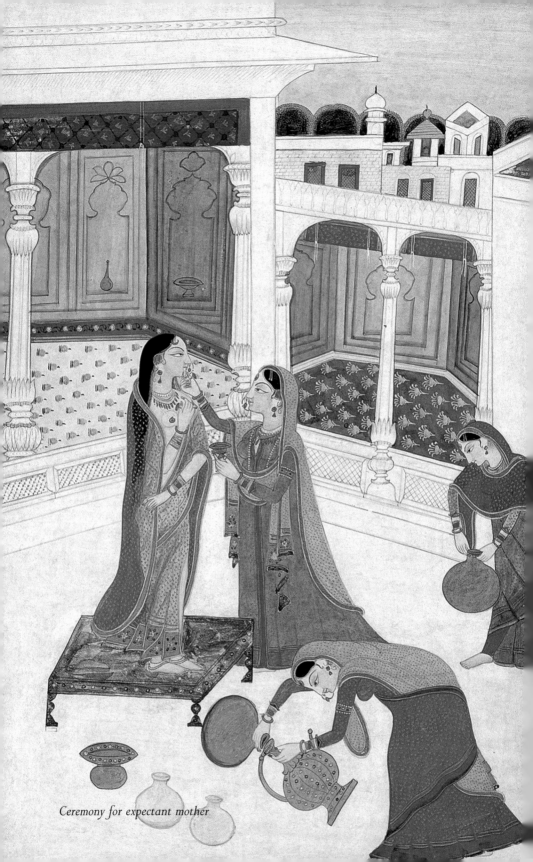

Ceremony for expectant mother

2.

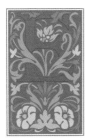

ve of Motherhood

"Your Miss Blake and her Major went off to Hampstead after their honeymoon," she wrote to me about the homecoming. Major McBride picked her up on the front porch and carried her over the threshold. That was all. Thereafter, they were cozy and happy living alone in their cottage. Of course, by then Miss Blake had made a regular practice of highlighting her hair with henna and cleansing her face with the almond saffron cream we made for her before she left.

But there the similarities in our lives ended. She was the sole mistress of her marriage and her life, whereas when I married, I entered the intricate web of joint family living. As the youngest daughter-in-law of the family I was mistress of very few things. It was my task to please everybody. To this day I am not sure of how many we were, all living together in that palace. My father-in-law, His Highness the Maharaja of Madanpur, had five important women living with him: two of his mothers and three wives. Then there were endless aunts, uncles, and cousins.

His Highness's mothers were retiring, quiet, and sweet. They rarely interfered in my life. But my mothers-in-law were a different story. We have a saying that goes: "She who has a good mother-in-law has the whole house; she who has a difficult mother-in-law cannot live long in the house." Fortunately, ours was a very big house, or I should say palace, so that made it easier to maintain good relations with three very different women.

Only one mother-in-law, of course, was really the mother of my beloved husband. She was Majli-Ma, the maharaja's second wife. They had an arranged marriage and she had borne her husband three children: a son, who was my husband's elder brother, then my husband, and last, a daughter. Majli-Ma was the religious one, always doing her *puja* and singing *bhajan* hymns. I admired her but did not know her well.

I was very close to my third mother-in-law, the one His Highness married for love. She was extremely affectionate and sweet natured. Chhoti-Ma was always chatting and laughing, doing a good turn for someone or cuddling one of the children. She had two daughters and two sons of her own, but of course, the daughters were married and gone.

It was the senior maharani, Badi-Ma, the first wife, who caused consternation. She was ten years older than His Highness, her husband, but everyone found this quite normal in an arranged royal marriage, even advantageous, as they openly said: "She stands an excellent chance of never being a widow, as she's sure to die before her husband."

always found that way of thinking hard to accept, but it didn't seem to trouble Badi-Ma at all. What troubled her was her childlessness. *Zenana* women felt that it was this shortcoming in life that provoked her sour disposition. We avoided her when at all possible, but the children of the palace adored her.

That is one nice thing about a joint family. Somehow every member finds his or her own special niche and is loved for a particular quality. Badi-Ma was a storehouse of myths, legends, and fairy tales. The children listened to her for hours. They never even seemed to notice that Badi-Ma "had salt in her skirt," as we say; she was hot-tempered, unpredictable, and she meddled in all our affairs. In a way it is wonderful for children to grow up with so many different people. It seems to make them more understanding, more outgoing, and less selfish. They learn to share at a very young age, and there is always someone to chat with or cuddle. They can depend on that. For that matter so could the grown-ups!

We relied on each other more than we knew, especially in times of crisis and sorrow, but also in times of great joy. Life was full of festivals and ceremonies in those days. Almost every month there was some big celebration.

How we preened ourselves preparing for them and how much we laughed together! This happened more in Madanpur than in my old home because we were so many more people.

All of those people were watching and waiting to see how soon I would conceive. But two years passed and I had nothing to announce. No one but Badi-Ma said anything but I knew what they were thinking: "A barren woman is a curse on the house, to see her face is to miss seven meals." I loved my husband and I was happy otherwise, so I tried to appear unconcerned.

Our daily routine left little time for brooding. Aside from celebrations and festivals, there were the evening *durbars* or open receptions held by my mothers-in-law in the *zenana*. Wives of noblemen and state officers would come and sit just to gossip and pass time. Sometimes women from the town came with complaints or special requests, which my mothers-in-law would look into. During the day there were the ritual *pujas* or religious observations; the supervision of meals, servants, and children; and of course, our own beauty care. Then, there was shopping.

Women of the town went to visit merchants in their shops. Palace women, though, could not go out often because of *purdah* restrictions, so the merchants came to see us in our quarters. There was the *bajaj* for all our fabric requirements, the *sonar* (goldsmith) for jewelry, the *gandhi* for perfumes and fragrant incense, and the *tamoli* for betel leaves. Surprisingly, our most important purveyor was the *pansari*, the local grocer. He did not come to us. We all gave him our orders through the household comptroller. He provided all the spices and herbs on which we depended for our various beauty treatments. It was the same with the *teli*, the oil vendor, whose fresh extractions we used for our hair, massage, home remedies, and of course, for the kitchen. All these merchants were crucial to our female fantasies, essential both for satisfying our vanity and for adding diversion to our days.

On the rare occasions when we went to Bombay, we were like children in our short-lived freedom. Escaping from *purdah*, we devoured the experience of shopping, eating in restaurants, and seeing cinemas. We would pretend to look quite worldly-wise in the shops as we stared at the strange bot-

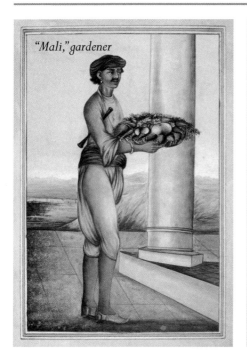

"Mali," gardener

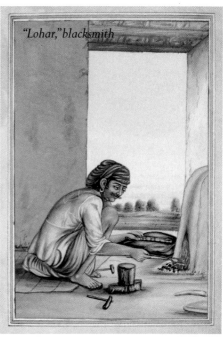

"Lohar," blacksmith

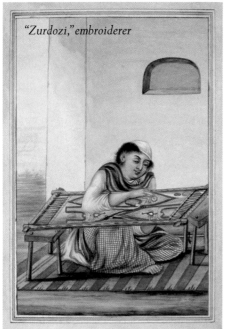

"Zurdozi," embroiderer

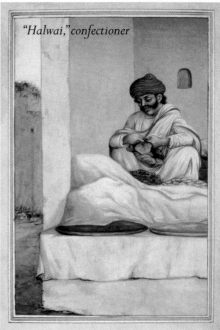

"Halwai," confectioner

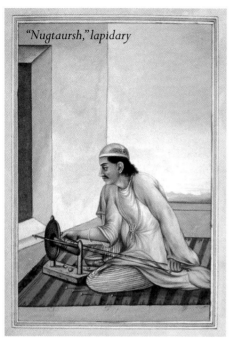

"Nugtaursh," lapidary

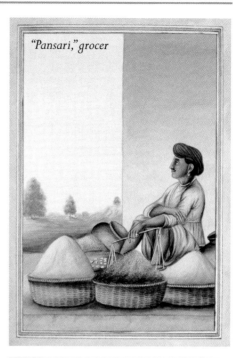

"Pansari," grocer

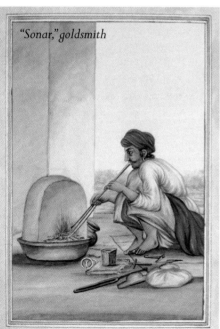

"Sonar," goldsmith

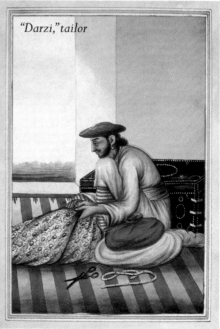

"Darzi," tailor

tled cosmetics. There was something called mascara, not unlike our *kaajal*; then there were creams and bright red lipsticks which only the courtesan dancers in Madanpur would dare to wear. How we laughed when my sister-in-law built up enough courage to purchase some cosmetics! I think they were Indian-made—something called Himalaya Snow, a sweet-smelling cold cream, and another called Desert Flower powder.

No one ever used them; we were far too familiar with the natural things we'd always used. But we loved the pictures on the labels—voluptuous women with their heads uncovered, smiling boldly with red lips and prominent breasts. Their hair was all loose like ours after a bath. They flaunted their freedom so openly. Those label pictures were a sort of western ideal of female liberation mixed with the Indian conception of beauty. No slim hips, flat chest, or short hair for that label lady! She was a real Indian Gauri in her proportions.

By Gauri I mean our favorite goddess, the wife of Lord Shiva, one of our most important deities. Gauri is an ideal beauty, like Padmini, but she is a goddess, not a human being. On Gangaur, which is Gauri's festival day, young unmarried girls pray that she finds them a good husband and married women ask her to protect their husbands, give them long life and marital bliss. There are many songs to Gauri. They speak of her sharp eyes and the lotus in her hands. Her head is fashioned like a coconut, her braid like a resplendent cobra, and her eyebrows like buzzing black bees.

Gauri's forehead is four fingers wide and her eyes sparkle like precious jewels. Her nose is sharp like a parrot's beak, her gums are like rubies, and her teeth dainty as pomegranate seeds. Her breasts are charmingly molded; her stomach is flat as a *peepal* leaf. Her feet are dainty as the lotus, but her thighs are firm and strong as temple pillars, and the heels of her feet shine like mirrors under her lovely skirt. So say all the songs about Gauri. We knew she wasn't real; that is, she was a goddess, but we thought Gauri was wonderful and we wanted to be like her. We considered her our ideal, our confidante, and friend. But I'm afraid Miss Blake did not understand. She had

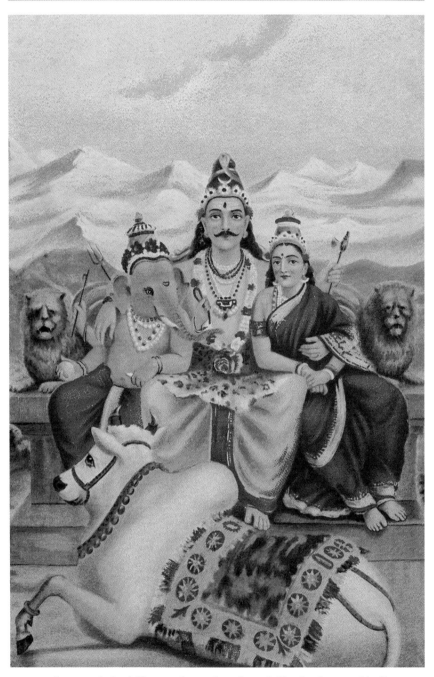

Gauri with Lord Shiva and son, Ganesh, with Nandi, the sacred bull

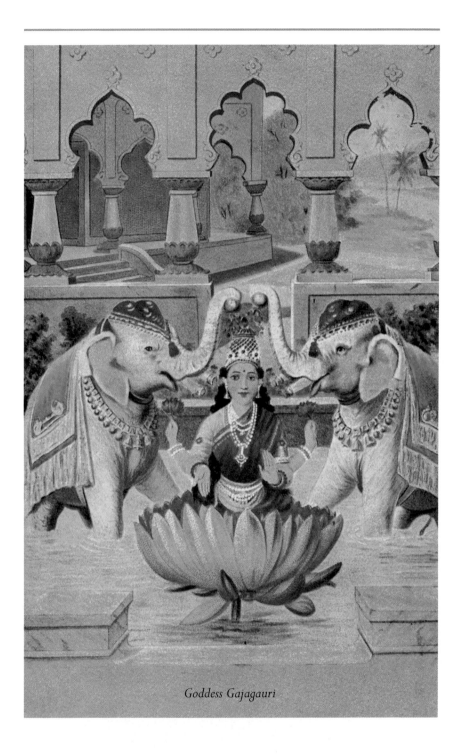

Goddess Gajagauri

little in common with that sort of beauty and Major McBride found it vulgar, I know, though he never would have said it out loud.

In my own heart, I began to pray to Gauri, not for a husband—I had a wonderful one—but for the child that did not seem to come. Badi-Ma, who had no children herself, was becoming ever so subtly cruel in her comments: "Padmini, didn't your own people teach you that family life is the best religion? We in Madanpur believe so." Perhaps she felt personally absolved of the crime of being childless because her co-wives had more than made up for her shortcoming? My real mother-in-law, busy with her *pujas*, said nothing outright, but frowned and sighed whenever she saw me, once or twice suggesting I might undertake fasts to appease the gods and speed up the child.

nly Chhoti-Ma, the youngest, left me in peace. When she saw me fasting and praying, she laughed, "Little Padmini, why on earth did God make males if women could conceive just by praying? Don't worry so. If the seed is strong and the earth is fertile, the crop will surely be bountiful. Your husband looks healthy and your periods are normal, so just relax, let nature take its course and I'm sure you'll spawn a whole cricket team!" I was so grateful to Chhoti-Ma for that. Her support carried me through the remaining months before my husband went off to Oxford. Then for two years the taunts and side glances ceased, I was left to my own devices while husband got his degree in England.

It was then that I turned to Pandit Dubey. He was by no means my lover, if that's what you're thinking. Pandit Dubey was a stout, scholarly man, almost eighty if he was a day, head of Madanpur State's Department of Religion, Astrology, and Ayurvedic Medicine. By this time in my life, thanks to Miss Blake's endless questions and my own experience with two *zenanas*, I had become very interested in that amorphous topic which is the subject of this book; beauty treatment, home remedies, and religious rites all rolled into one. Pandit Dubey was a master in this field.

Pandit means "a learned man." Pandit Dubey was a *Raj Vaid*, the royal ayurvedic doctor, astrologer, and guide, whose portfolio was our health, our general well-being, and the success of the Madanpur line. I talked to him of these matters for hours. Looking back, I'm sure that many of my questions must have amused him. Much of what he told me was hard to follow, especially the basis of ayurvedic medicine.

According to ayurveda, human beings are a blend of three component elements: air and space, which is called *vatam;* earth and water, which is *kapham;* and energy and water, which is *pittam*. If the three are in equilibrium, a person is healthy; if not, he will always be ill. The ultimate aim of ayurveda is to restore and maintain this balance. As each person's constitution is unique, so the treatment is highly individual and specific, tailored to one's psyche, environment, diet, symptoms, and age. The same treatment, which succeeds with one patient, may totally fail with another, though the two patients may have the very same symptoms.

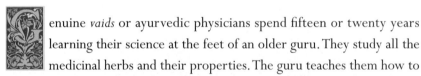enuine *vaids* or ayurvedic physicians spend fifteen or twenty years learning their science at the feet of an older guru. They study all the medicinal herbs and their properties. The guru teaches them how to distill their own herbal formulas in earthen vessels. He also specifies the particular season and phase of the moon when each medicinal plant or herb is to be plucked and distilled. The students learn to reduce precious metals, gems, and shells to ashes in specially built furnaces. All this alchemy is done in the interest of science, particularly the art of healing. As I sat enthralled behind my small *purdah* screen, Pandit Dubey told me much of these wonders.

Together we read famous medical texts like *Sushruta* and *Charak Samhita,* very serious, erudite works. But Panditji was familiar with folk medicine, too. The little stepdaughter of ayurveda, folk medicine has been practiced in India forever. In fact, we still use it today.

Chhoti-Ma gave me one such folk remedy when she heard that my husband was returning from England. She learned this remedy from her grandmother, but Pandit Dubey said it was well known in ayurveda and suggested that I try it. In those days no one had heard of fertility drugs. We just knew that certain herbs and spices and plants had properties that "heated" or "cooled" the body. That did not mean heated or cooled like a fan; it increased or decreased the "internal fires," those elements of *kapham, vatam, pittam* that had to be kept in balance.

I took the potion made of new banyan shoots from Chhoti-Ma and, sure enough, they stoked some internal fires, for within a month of my husband's return, I was expecting a baby! Chhoti-Ma later told me how to make that potion: pluck the tender, new shoots of the banyan tree, grind them, and form them into marble-sized pellets. Then take one in the morning and one in the evening for four days after your period is over. Somehow it pleased me to be so indebted to the tree I had loved as a child, the friendly banyan with its tentacle trunks and myriad branches, which I used to swing on for hours.

There was much rejoicing in the palace when my condition became common knowledge. The news spread very fast although, technically speaking, such delicate matters are never discussed openly. I paid no attention to who knew or how they had learned. I was much too happy to worry about how people found out and too busy to care. Expectant mothers in our country have a lot of good advice to follow and many rituals to perform.

Conception is an extremely important stepping stone in the Hindu scheme of human progression. It is the first of sixteen *sanskars* or sacred rites every Hindu must observe as she progresses through life. Ten of those *sanskars*, in fact, take place between conception and the child's first solid feeding. *Sanskars* are taken very seriously, especially by the likes of Pandit Dubey. Because they involve elements of religion, education, hygiene, and tradition, they are a must for every orthodox Hindu.

I can now admit that I did not clearly understand the philosophy, but I happily performed all the rites. Even the first one, *garbhadaan* or conception, was subject to the Pandit's approval. In his role as royal astrologer, Pandit Dubey had chosen not only the auspicious day, but also the auspicious moment for conception, according to the position of the stars, moon, and planets! My husband and I laughed about this later as we held our sweet baby, but before her birth there were four other *sanskars*. Of these I particularly remember one called *anavalobhan* that takes place in the third month of preg-

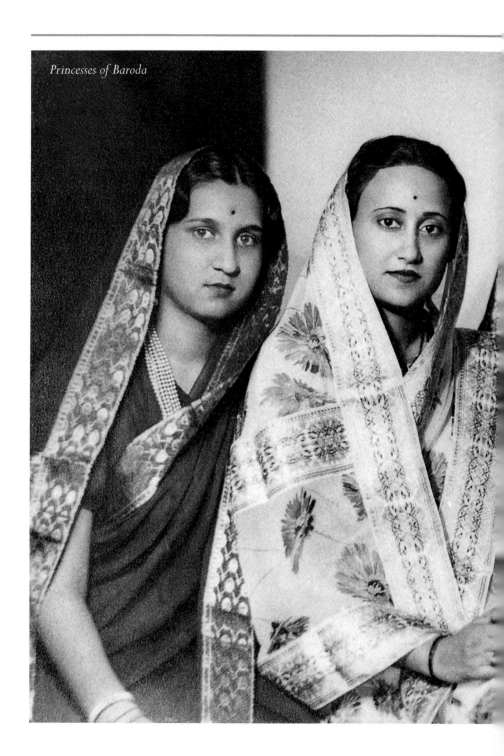

Princesses of Baroda

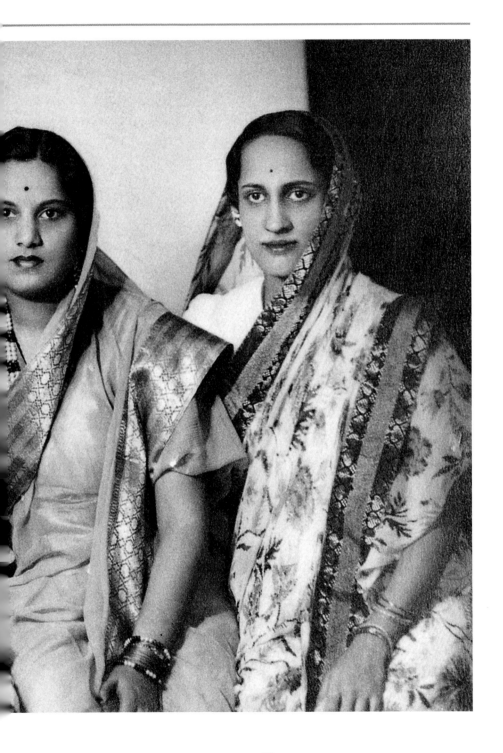

nancy. For that ritual my husband put two drops of juice from the sacred *durva* grass into my right nostril, to ensure the well being of the child. *Durva* grass is the common *harialee* or *dub* grass, used in Hindu ceremonies. All I know is that it tickled and I tried very hard not sneeze!

The moment people knew that I was expecting, everyone had some suggestion to make, from the Pandit to my shyest little maid. I began to realize that Indians really believe that beauty treatments begin in the womb. Even old senior grandmother contributed. She came out of her retreat to bring me a spoon of ground almonds in a glass of hot milk every single night for nine months. She assured me that this simple potion would make my little one very fair. I know she meant well but I winced at this accent on skin color.

Miss Blake had admired our golden complexions and had opened my eyes to that beauty. But the rest of India wanted pale complexions, the less wheaten the better. Pandit Dubey even whispered an old Sanskrit couplet to me; it meant that the color of the food consumed by the mother affects the color of the child in her womb! So I kept quiet and took everyone's advice, even my mother's. She wrote to say I must add a teaspoon of turmeric powder to my milk every day—again in the interest of fairness.

Then middle mother-in-law took time off from her *pujas* to tell me that I must add not only a teaspoonful of turmeric, but also a tiny pinch of saffron to the milk, this time not in the interest of fairness but to ensure an easy labor. The glass, she added, must be of silver because of its cooling properties. Many people believe that metals affect whatever they touch and that they are "heating" or "cooling," beneficial or harmful, auspicious or inauspicious, according to their composition. All I know is that my child was born with a lovely complexion and perhaps because of the turmeric and saffron in my milk, I never caught a cold those nine months.

Through the years, I have chatted with women from so many places, to learn about their traditions. An old friend from Bengal, in eastern India, whose husband had settled in Madanpur, told me her people had the same

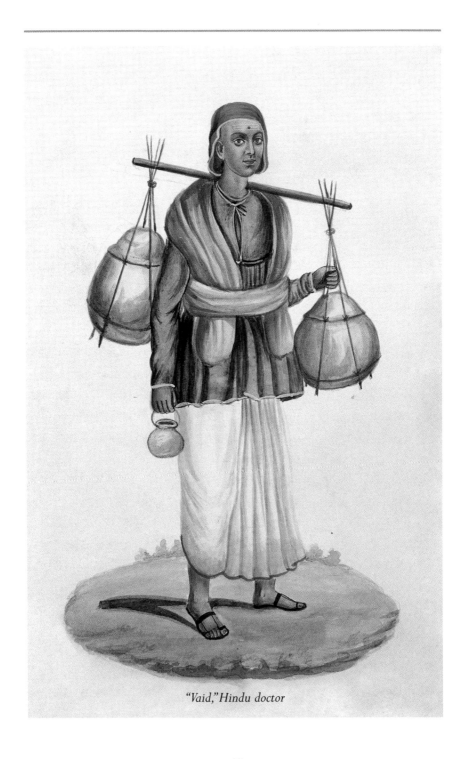

"Vaid," Hindu doctor

obsession with fairness, only they made her drink coconut water instead of almonds and milk when she was expecting a child. Bengal has coconuts; we in Rajasthan had almonds brought from the north by traders. Ideas and traditions spring from the readily available. The white color of almonds, cashews, and coconuts must have appealed to women and therefore gave them hopes about fairness and slowly such ideas became rules.

I don't believe there's more to the theory than that; but the same Bengali friend who told me of coconut for fairness also told me about hair. I felt those hair theories of hers might have more substance. She said Bengali women make a point of eating greens throughout pregnancy because they ensure a thick growth of hair for the child. She even gave me a recipe for delicious mixed greens, which I sent to Miss Blake, when she was expecting. Miss Blake, or I should say, Mrs. McBride, always admired our long, thick, black hair and said how much she feared having bald babies.

So she sat in Hampstead expecting her first child and made this dish, called *chachchari*: Wash and trim about 250 grams (½ pound) of your favorite greens. Set them aside next to the stove after chopping them very fine. You will need about 2 cups of chopped greens. Mix together ½ teaspoon each of the following spice seeds and also keep them close to the stove: fenugreek, cumin, aniseed, black mustard, and bishop's weed (*ajwain*). Bengalis call this spice mix *panch phoron*, five condiments.

Heat 2 tablespoons of any cooking oil in a shallow skillet. Keep its lid close by the stove. When the oil starts smoking, toss in the spices, and quickly put the lid on the skillet. Shake it about until the seeds start to sputter, then take off the lid and stir in the greens. Cook them over high heat until wilted.

have never met Miss Blake's little girl, but the photograph of her when she got married showed a splendid head of dark chestnut hair. Be that as it may, I've got ahead of myself. I was still expecting a baby until I got sidetracked with spinach and fenugreek leaves! Such things were very far from my mind in those very first days of my pregnancy. I couldn't

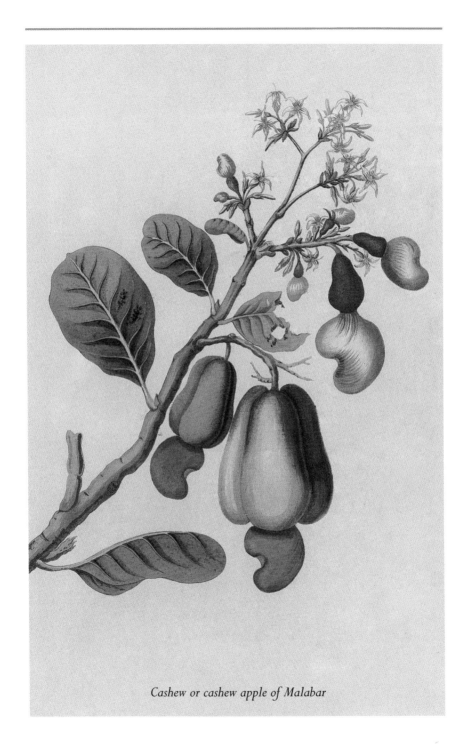

Cashew or cashew apple of Malabar

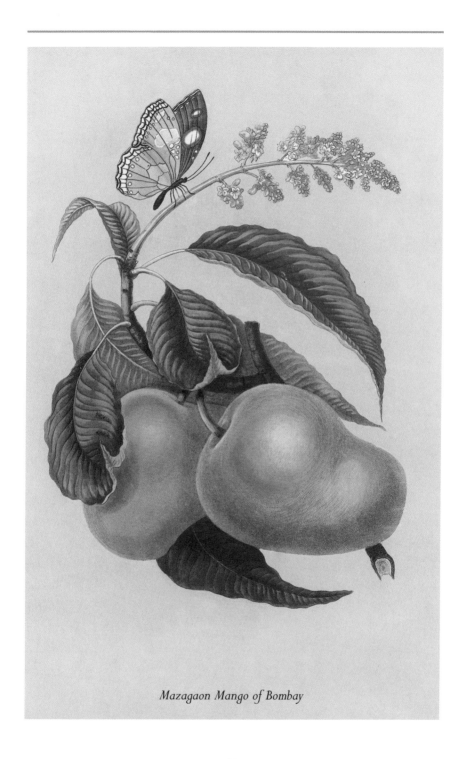

Mazagaon Mango of Bombay

even drink tea, let alone think of food! Everything made me feel sick, until Chhoti-Ma again came to the rescue with several folk remedies, these too from her old grandmother. I could either drink basil leaf tea, she suggested, or I could chew roasted cloves and cardamoms or I might try spicing my milk with a bit of rock candy and an extract of fresh ginger juice. The ginger juice worked! My morning sickness was cured. At last I understood a saying I'd heard: "Only four days married and she's off to the grocer's to buy herself a stock of ginger." It hadn't made sense until then.

There were so many do's and don'ts to consider. My maids were told to no longer give me massages with perfumed oils or abrasive concoctions like the *peethi* they had rubbed at my wedding. In my condition massage was forbidden. But mother wrote to me about the exercise I should do to make my muscles supple for the confinement. Although a princess was not expected to perform menial tasks, she advised me to do two, which she had done herself from the third month through to the end of her six confinements. First of all she suggested that I should sit on the floor and grind at the stone hand-mill for fifteen minutes every day. This would strengthen my spine and back and make them flexible she said. The other task was to churn butter the traditional Indian way. Sour cream and cold water are put into a large earthen pot and churned with a long wooden churn-staff which is tied to the wall. Mother said the action of pulling back and forth the two ends of the cord that is entwined around the staff would also strengthen the spine and develop the muscles that support the growing breasts.

I had to follow a very strict dietary regime. In the first and second months of pregnancy, I was to eat only cereals which grow in sixty days, like rice. In the first three months, the cereals were mixed with milk, then in the fourth month with yogurt, with milk again in the fifth month, and in the sixth month mixed with clarified butter. I do not know why this was done.

oods like papayas and pineapples, which I loved, were taboo because according to the women of the *zenana*, their "heating" properties could cause a miscarriage. I was encouraged to eat plenty of other fruits, but all fried, spicy, and sour foods were forbidden as they cause indigestion, by the *zenana* way of thinking.

"May you bathe in milk and be fruitful in children" was one of Pandit Dubey's favorite benedictions. I always thought it very sweet too, but by my fifth or sixth month I began to dread milk, I felt I was drowning in it! So many relatives dropped in solicitously to offer me a little glass of— guess what? In the seventh month, it became twice a day. Every morning I had to drink a glass of milk mixed with clarified butter. Everyone said that made childbirth easy. In any case, Indians seem to have a mania about clarified butter, which is called *ghee*. "Neither mother nor father can do as much good as *ghee*," we say. All I know is that milk became a sort of obsession. To top it all off, in my eighth and ninth months, I was told to reduce my intake of all other foods and increase my consumption of milk!

Practically afloat in dairy products, I spent my days reading religious books and listening to soft, soothing *bhajans,* our songs or prayers, which are so lovely. My husband insisted that I stay in his home for the child's delivery. Normally girls return to their mothers in the sixth month, at least for the birth of the first child. As I did not, mother wrote continuously, stressing the importance of my attitude. Just as she had told me many years before, that "a good nature makes a good face," now she wrote to say I must stay happy and calm, not quarrel or even get angry.

We believe all these things affect the child in the womb. And we believe in telling that child stories while he's in his mother's tummy. I remember one about a Rajput warrior, which is so typical of our concept of honor: it was about a warrior who ran from a battle and returned home to his wife. Mortified by her husband's conduct, she sent him to ask his mother how she could have produced such a coward.

"Something is amiss here," said the mother, furious with shame for her son. "Any child who has drunk my milk will either die fighting or come home victorious." Then she interrogated all of her maids and found the answer to her son's cowardice. It seems one of her maids had secretly

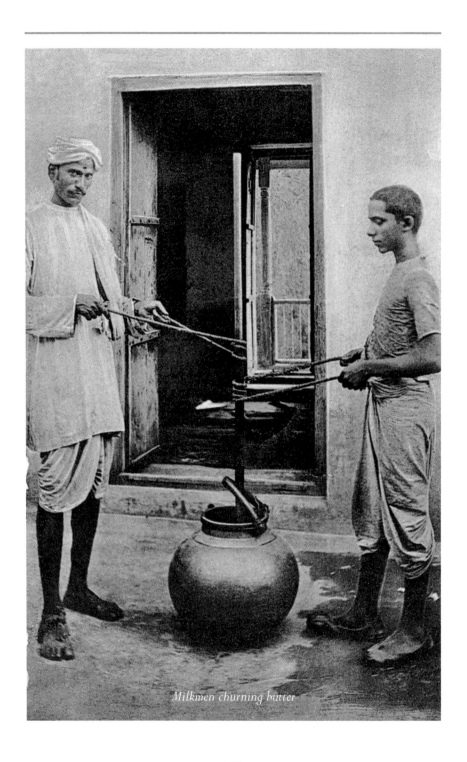

Milkmen churning butter

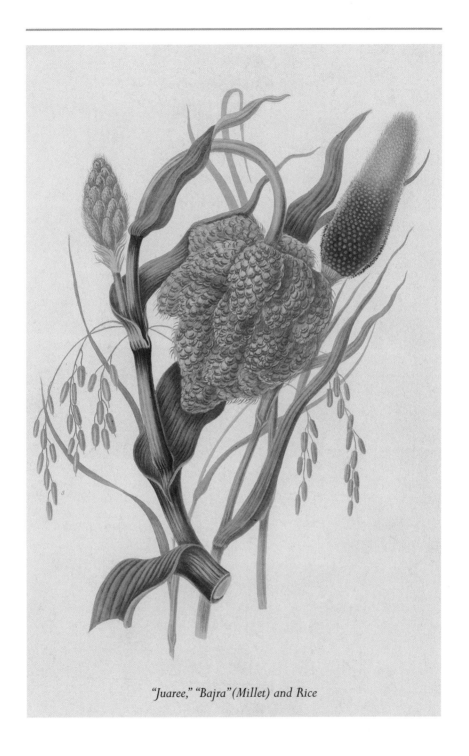

"Juaree," "Bajra"(Millet) and Rice

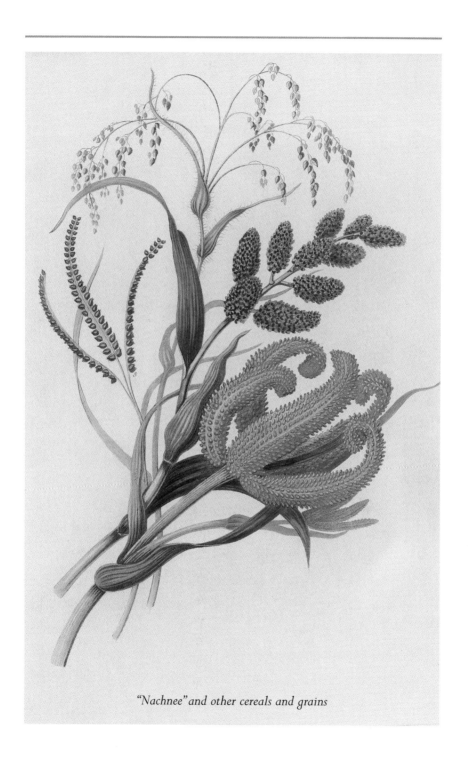

"Nachnee" and other cereals and grains

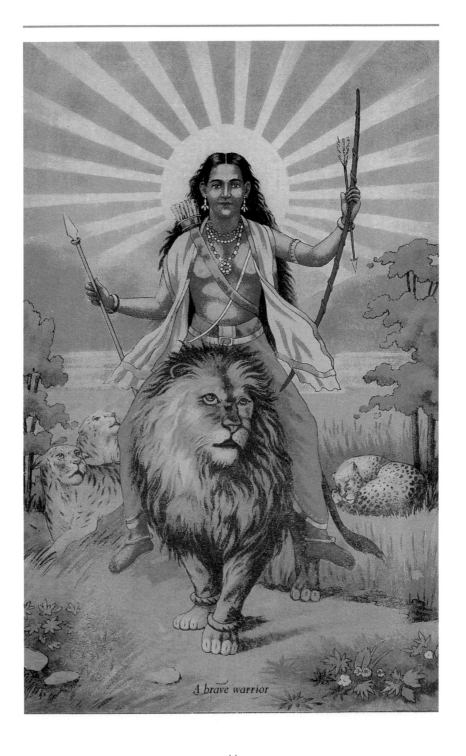

A brave warrior

suckled the boy with her own milk on one occasion when he cried and his mother was not there.

The moral of the story? According to the bards who used to sing us such tales, one has to be very careful who looks after one's child. Her character will influence the child, just like this maid's milk made the baby a coward!

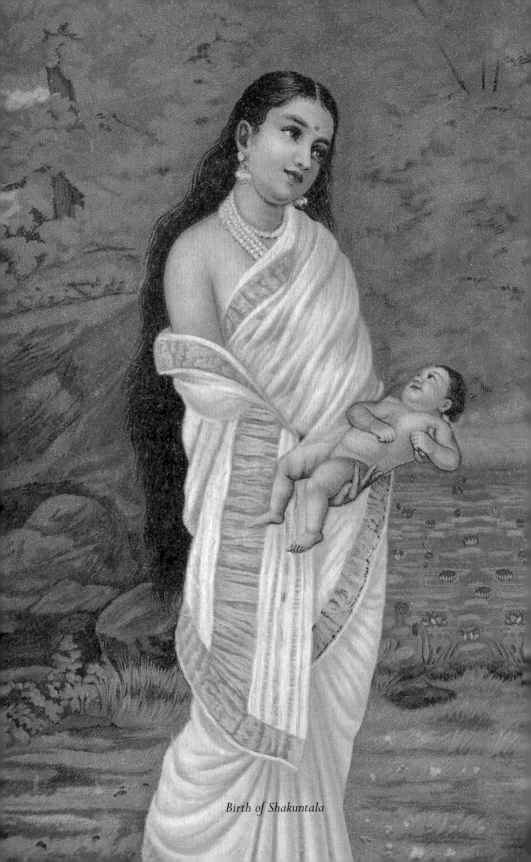

Birth of Shakuntala

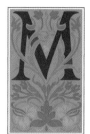

aternal Joys

Though I may not have had full faith in that story, I chose my baby's nurse with great care. She was soft-spoken, kind, and deeply religious. Her own children were quite well brought up. Like all royal nursemaids, she was given the title of Dai-Ma, nurse mother. She had a special status in the *zenana* and was treated with respect and honor. I don't think Dai-Ma minded that my child was a daughter. She was there when the baby was born. After all the fuss, it was an easy delivery. Pandit Dubey had prescribed a small cup of warm clarified butter just after the baby emerged. This, he said, would hasten the placenta and prevent the pain of the uterus contracting, even bring it back to normal more quickly. I hardly remember any of that; I only had eyes for my baby.

Dai-Ma wrapped her and took her from me. I remember thinking, "now somebody else will have to drink milk for a while!"

The palace made a brave show of celebration, even though they'd wanted a son. Sweets were distributed, and according to custom the palace women all came to sing. That is our tradition in Rajasthan; for five weeks the women come and sing to the mother, morning and evening. Sweet songs, they were meant to entertain me and break the monotony of my confinement; but they were all about the *jachcha*, our word for mother, and her adorable son!

"Our lovely *jachcha* queen is like the *peepal* tree," they sang. "Her branches now laden with fruit. She gave birth to her son in the dark of the night; in the morning with great joy, we sent sweet brown sugar to announce his arrival to the world. Now she is tired, resting in her bed, a goddess being fanned by her maids. Her silver boxes, filled with lampblack, overflow with good fortune…" and so on. I sometimes fell asleep while they sang.

Confinement was not as simple as I'd expected. I should perhaps explain that in India a woman is considered unclean, in a ritual sense, for ten days among the Hindus and forty among the Muslims, after the baby is born. She must remain apart from other people, just like a menstruating woman. Among certain people, only the midwife and other special attendants can visit her during this time. It seems a harsh rule, but I suppose it also serves a purpose, forcing a woman to rest in peace until she can regain her strength.

e strongly believe that rest is important. If a woman does not take proper care of herself after the baby is born, she will suffer later with back problems, sagging stomach, and chronic weakness. Village women must be especially careful; they have so much hard work to do the moment their confinement is over. But in my time, all women, rich and poor used to follow a strict regimen of diet and massage after their babies were born. The techniques and the food varied with the region and the climate where the child was born, but there was always strong emphasis on shrinking the stomach, strengthening the back, and increasing the mother's breast milk.

While Dai-Ma looked after my baby girl and brought her to me for feedings, Jijabai the massage woman took me in her charge and looked after me for two months. She was a real martinet, but she had the most wonderful, loving, and experienced hands; she had cared for so many women. I had a strict routine. For one hour every morning, Jijabai would massage me. Starting with my stomach, she worked very, very gently, always rubbing in a clockwise direction, never lifting her hands from my body. For the rest of the body, she pressed hard towards the heart, then drew back gently in the other direction.

For the back massage she didn't press the spinal cord at all, just placed her thumbs on either side of it and went hard upward and gently downward. Jijabai was not from Rajasthan, though she'd spent many years in the

Madanpur palace; she was a Maharashtrian from south of Bombay and her methods were all from that region.

The oil she used for massage contained powdered mango-ginger, a variety of turmeric we call *ambia haldi*, which is *Curcuma amada* in Latin; it also contained ground bitter gourd, a vegetable we call *karela*. These two ingredients are known to prevent itching, rashes or skin allergies.

The massage was always followed by a *dhoori*. Miss Blake was quite amazed by this procedure when I wrote to her about it. You see, I had to seat myself on a cot, which I described to Miss Blake as something like her old garden chair. It had webbing for a bottom, so you saw the floor through it. Underneath the cot burned a little coal fire. And on that fire Jijabai put a powder she prepared every morning.

Pandit Dubey explained to me the English and Latin equivalents of the ingredients she put in the powder. There were garlic peel; *ajwain* or bishop's weed; *balant shepa* seeds or dill; and *wowding* seeds that, according to the Pandit, are fruit of *Embelia ribes*. They look like small black pepper pods when they're dry; but Miss Blake could not identify them from my description, so perhaps they are not found outside India.

Jijabai would put a tiny sprinkling of this powder on the coals and the fragrance would waft up through the cot webbing on to my exposed "'nether parts," as dear Miss Blake always called them. The smoke really helps to contract the vagina and the uterus so they return to normal as soon as possible. Many women in Rajasthan and elsewhere in India use this or other similar methods.

Some substitute dried cow dung for the coal and dried powder I used. That surprises many people, but Hindus believe that all products of the cow—milk, yogurt, clarified butter, urine, and even dung—are pure, sacred, and beneficial. I know that's offensive to some people. It was to me, too, until a doctor I know said there could be some truth in it all. He said research had confirmed that the use of cow dung as flooring and plaster in many Indian villages might well be responsible for the fact that the incidence of tuberculosis in rural conditions is lower than might be expected. It seems cow dung may really be antiseptic.

Jijabai also prepared a medicinal douche by boiling together alum, *khadir* (also called *kaat, kathha,* or *khair* which we use in *paan* and is known in Latin as *Acacia catechu*), and bark of the *babul* tree which is *Acacia arabica*. I would dilute the concentrated solution with water and wash my "nether parts," again to contract them as quickly as possible. All three are astringents and these prevented itching. Jijabai suggested that I should use the same diluted solution for gargling. After childbirth, she said, the teeth become weak and this would help to strengthen the gums and prevent tooth decay.

I was so young then that I didn't question all these things. I just did what the elders advised. When I went to my mother for my second confinement, I even sat in a tub of water to which *aasha*, a local Rajasthani spirit, had been added. Thirty-two herbal ingredients had been soaked for fifteen days in that *aasha*. This procedure was intended to reduce my body's water retention and encourage all the organs to contract. Not only did I have to sit in that *aasha*, I also had to drink it on the tenth day after childbirth, mixed with a cup of clarified butter. My mother's maid swore this helped the uterus to contract normally without any pain.

Indian midwives are particularly keen on this business of contracting organs. Today, in Bombay, I have a Muslim masseuse who comes from the coast, south of Bombay. Of course, there is no further question of contracting my organs, but she and I like to chitchat.

She told me about an herbal remedy, handed down to her from her mother and grandmother. To make it, she steams two handfuls of tamarind seeds and puts them to dry in the sun. When the outer skin dries and peels, she pounds these seeds and sieves the powder. To this she adds turmeric powder, a little brandy, and some raw sugar, and kneads it all together to make long, slender pellets. She wraps the pellets in a sterilized piece of muslin, making a sort of village tampon. A length of string is left to protrude and the rest is inserted into the vagina, right up to the cervix where it remains overnight, to be removed in the morning.

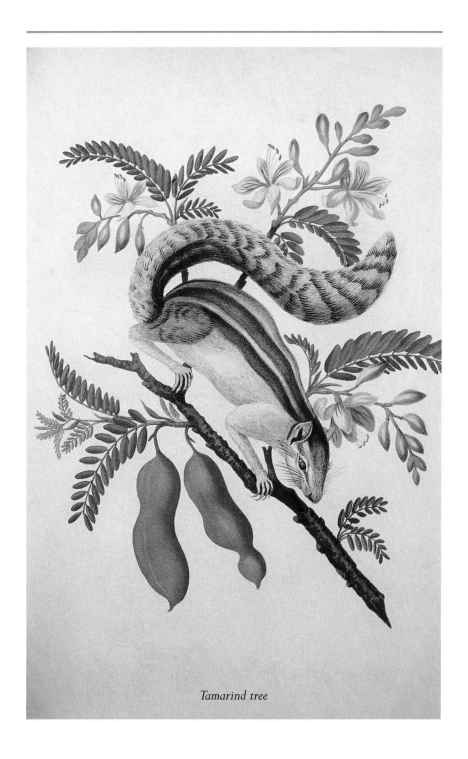

Tamarind tree

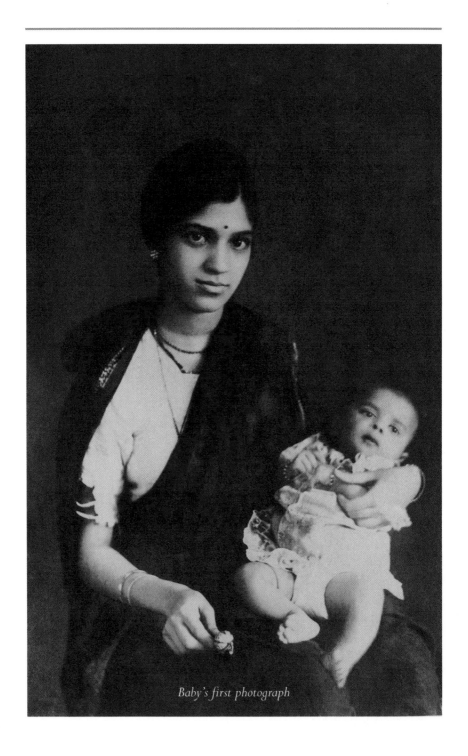

Baby's first photograph

My massage woman does this for three days if the patient only wants "her vagina to be like a virgin," for seven days if she does not want to conceive for another two or three years, and for fifteen days if she has decided that she doesn't want any more children.

I would never try such things, though I love to hear about them. There must surely be a danger of infection. In fact this whole idea of contraception is something women discussed with reluctance, even when we were alone. I do not know much about it. I've been told there are women in the northwest frontier, near the Khyber Pass, who have a wonderful knowledge of many roots and herbs, and who make little contraceptive tablets to be inserted into the vagina. I don't know anyone who has actually used these. For the most part, I suppose we just relied on breastfeeding our children as long as we could to avoid conception. Then we left the rest to our gods.

Now, I've gone very astray from my "smoking" procedure! After I'd sat on that cot for a while, letting the smoke do its work, it was time for a bath. I was as regimented in those days as my sweet little daughter; though she was getting more sleep than I!

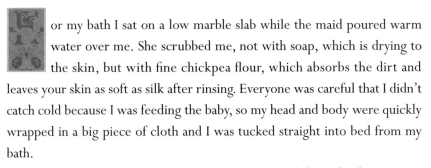or my bath I sat on a low marble slab while the maid poured warm water over me. She scrubbed me, not with soap, which is drying to the skin, but with fine chickpea flour, which absorbs the dirt and leaves your skin as soft as silk after rinsing. Everyone was careful that I didn't catch cold because I was feeding the baby, so my head and body were quickly wrapped in a big piece of cloth and I was tucked straight into bed from my bath.

There the maid would tie my stomach very tightly with a long cotton *sari*. This went on for forty days! I never liked that old Indian corset; but it kept my stomach flat and supported my back, and I have never had any trouble with either, even though now I have put on a little weight here in Bombay. It was heavenly lying there all warm and clean in my bed. Dai-Ma would bring the little one for feeding and my husband would sneak in to chat for a while as she drank her fill. The *zenana* ladies were scandalized at his being there and being so attentive. While he told me all the news of the palace, someone would light a little brazier under my bed and throw sandal-wood shavings or incense on it so the smoke would keep insects away and the fire would warm my back after the bath. Before I knew it, I would drop off to sleep and Dai-Ma would take the baby.

Chhoti-Ma, the youngest mother-in-law, was very proud of her little granddaughter. She used to say that one of the nicest things about a new baby was the good food prepared for the mother! That is true, but in my case, not until the tenth day after the birth of the baby.

For the first three days after I delivered, I was not even given water to drink. My women explained that that was because water prevented the abdominal muscles from contracting. I had to go along with this contracting business, so for those three days I drank only plain milk, milk with a little coffee, and *sooji ki kheer,* which is semolina cooked in milk and sugar. Then for a week, I ate cooked fenugreek leaves with millet bread, our favorite *bajri ki roti.* We all believe that millet is very "heating" to one's "internal fires." My maids assured me it was extremely helpful in emptying the uterus of blood that remained there after the delivery.

n the tenth day came the sweet preparations Chhoti-Ma was refer-ring to—the best thing about having a baby! There was a simple one of semolina, clarified butter, and sugar called *halwa* and another called *katloo*, made from no less than forty-four ingredients. I never learned them all, but I know there was wheat flour, gum arabic, chickpeas, dried fruits, pumpkin seeds, and clarified butter. All forty-four ingredients were first roasted and pounded, then mixed together with raw brown sugar and shaped into balls.

These *katloo* balls were first ritually offered to the family deity, then they were given to me. I was ordered to eat a whole kilo of *katloos* within the next thirty days! They were believed by one and all to be generally strengthening as well as good inducers of milk. For the matter of my milk, there were several little jars on my bedside table, each containing some-

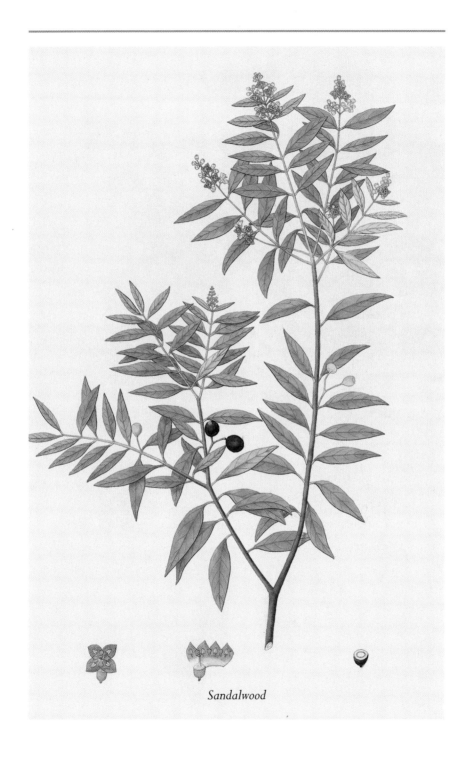

Sandalwood

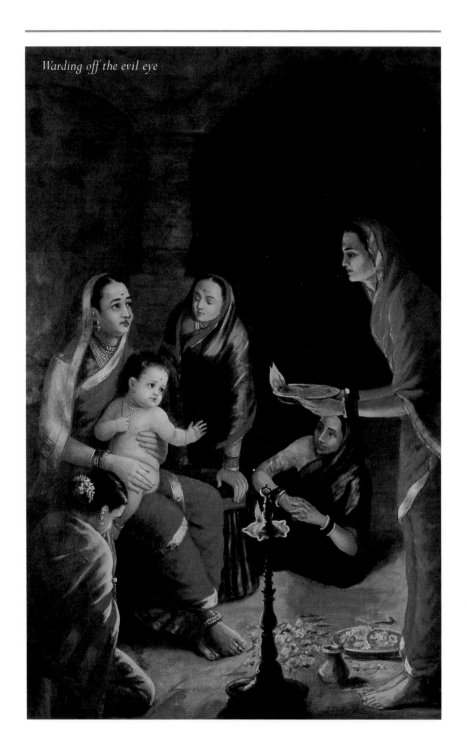

Warding off the evil eye

thing someone believed to be milk inducing. There were dry flakes of coconut; *balant shepa* (dill) seeds which, according to the Pandit, were eaten to purify the breast milk; little sweet balls made of *ahliv* (common cress seeds); and occasionally a curry of *arvi* leaves, *Colocasia antiquorum* in Latin. Imagine that word on a menu!

Badi-Ma, of all people, brought me a measure of salted *ajwain*, bishop's weed or caraway seeds, tucked in a tiny silver box. She said they should be chewed to prevent indigestion, which might upset the baby's tummy, too. When I went home for my second confinement, mother made me a brew called *dasmool*, made from the roots of ten medicinal plants, which she said was very good for inducing milk.

One maid told me that in her village, when a mother's breasts are overly full, they put a fomentation of warm leaves from the castor oil plant. I never had that problem but I did have enough milk to feed my little child for nine months and I was quite proud of that. Just like the maids with their little ones, I would sit cross-legged with my baby in my lap. Hugging her close, I would automatically cover her whole body with the end of my *odhni* scarf to shield her from the evil eye. Though I knew better, I couldn't help it.

he evil eye is probably something everyone in this country is aware of, though they may not believe in it. I've found very little else we all have in common. It's such a big and diverse country. For example, look at the difference in diet for a mother. Mine was light for the first ten days, but a Brahmin friend from Kashmir told me of her diet that was the exact opposite. For the first ten days of their confinement, women of her community in Kashmir are fed rich, fried breads called *parathas* cooked in clarified butter and eaten with grilled meat or liver that's been seasoned with black pepper and dried ginger powder. After the tenth day, milk is added to that diet, along with a meat soup called *shorba,* and a thick semolina pudding. You could only eat such foods in Kashmir's cold climate. In Madanpur, I would have expired!

Where the climate is hot in south India, the regimen is different from the heavy meat diet of Kashmir. The accent is on leafy green vegetables which cause no problem with the mother's digestion. Vegetables like potatoes and cauliflower are avoided because they cause gas; also pumpkin because it can cause rashes on the baby's body, or so we believe.

In south India the emphasis is not only on what you eat, but also on the sequence of the meal. They feel it is important, from a health point of view, to eat different flavors, textures, and types of food in the appropriate order. My friend told me that during her confinement she always began her meal with two handfuls of hot rice. The rice was mixed with hot clarified butter, powdered cumin, and black peppercorns that had been fried and then ground. All those ingredients are considered "heating."

According to my friend, they prevented her from catching a cold or cough throughout the time she fed the baby. She also took a lot of the family's favorite home remedy, *leghyam*. *Leghyam* is a sort of herbal cure-all that her mother made from forty different herbs and spices that she kept stored in a tightly sealed bottle. The first thing she would eat in the morning during her confinement was a teaspoon of *leghyam* that had been premixed with a handful of fried garlic pods.

This business of garlic seems to be common in India. In Goa, confined mothers drink garlic soup, *lasun ki kadhi*, both to reduce gas and to induce breast milk. I've had it once; it's made of garlic, coconut, chilies, and *kokam*, a local sour fruit, and it's absolutely delicious.

It's strange that so many of the foods we consider beneficial seem to be either very sour, bitter, or extremely pungent. In fact, one of our old proverbs advises us to "eat bitter foods at least once a week and sweets only once a month" to keep good health. I cannot imagine that any other nation eats more garlic than we do. "Garlic is as good as ten mothers," we say. Mind you, it is almost always cooked in such a way that its flavor marries with many others and its smell never comes on one's breath. Indians think garlic is good for everything: digestion, complexion, night blindness, even for mend-

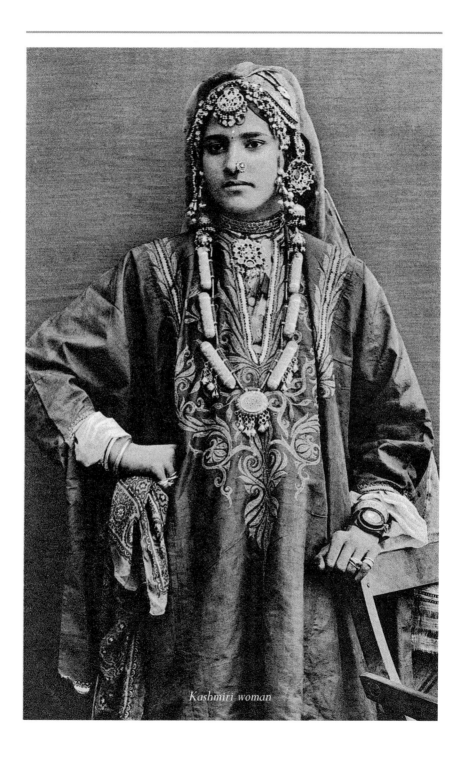

Kashmiri woman

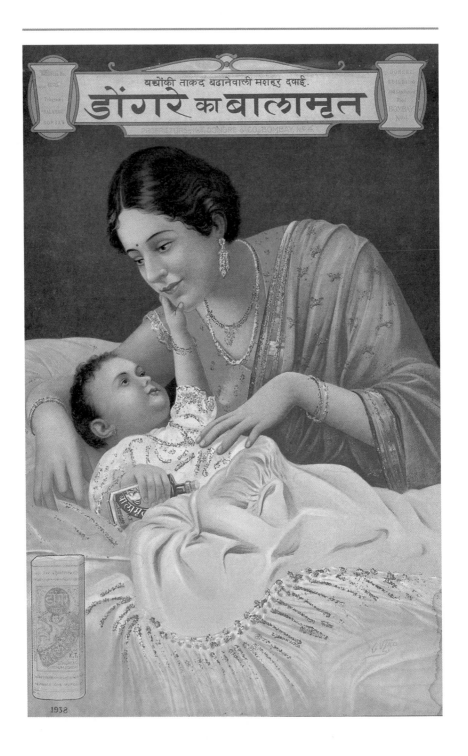

ing broken bones and sharpening the intellect. If that were true, we should be the brightest people on earth! In any case, we go on hopefully ingesting it, beginning with our own mother's milk. My massage woman urged me to use garlic for a purpose I would never have imagined! She would boil a handful of garlic pods in coconut oil until they turned pink, then strain this oil and give it to me to apply on my "nether parts"! She assured me this oil would prevent infection and the itching we all suffer after childbirth when this area becomes a bit dry.

y the time I had my third child, I had heard of a hundred home remedies and secrets for new mothers and babies. Among the many I had tried, some were strange and seemed useless, but many were delicious, just as Chhoti-Ma had remarked. My three favorites were sweets, of course, two from Maharashtra and one from the Punjab, in north India, sent by a very dear Sikh friend of my mother's. It was called *panjiri*; and it was intended to give strength and to produce more milk in the lactating mother. Just like *katloo*, it contained dried fruits, almonds, and pistachios, but it also had semolina, black pepper, gum arabic, and *phool-makana* made from the dried root of the lotus. All of this was mixed with sugar and clarified butter and, like *katloo*, made into little balls.

The ones from Maharashtra were brought by Jijabai, my massage woman. One was bitter, but somehow I liked it. It was prepared with roasted fenugreek seeds and melted sugar syrup and made into little balls. The other was made from gum arabic, which I believe is rich in calcium and calcium salts and is therefore very good for the back. The gum arabic was fried and mixed with wonderful things like sugar, musk, saffron, dried ginger, clove, black pepper, cardamom, nutmeg, dried fruit, coconut, and poppy seeds.

I often wondered how many people and how many hours it took to prepare such delights. Those hours and those people seem to be disappearing now, and with them all these old remedies.

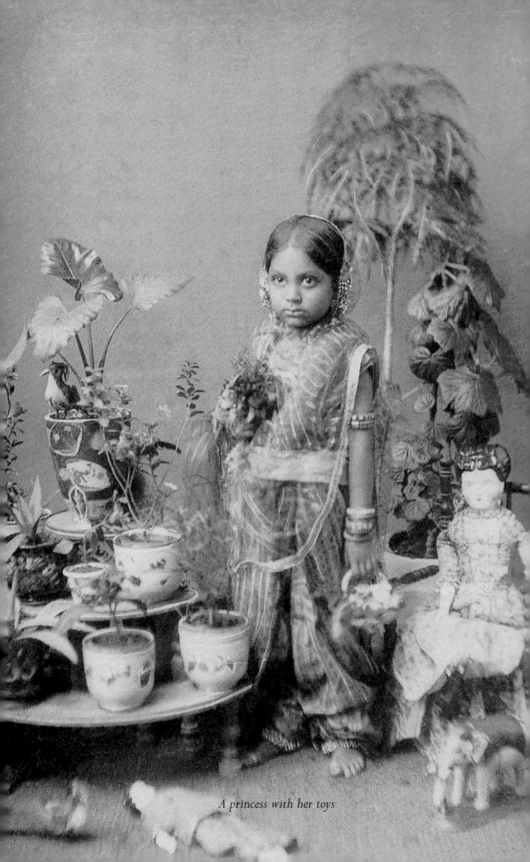

A princess with her toys

4.

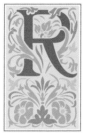

Raising a Family

Thank goodness all those people with hours to spare had not disappeared during the period when I was raising my family; they all contributed so much to the flavor of our lives and to the character of my children. The two most influential ones were, of course, Dai-Ma their nurse, and Pandit Dubey, my mentor in everything from religion to folklore.

It was Pandit Dubey who whispered in my ear after my second daughter was about two years old that we might try a little trick he knew of; that is, if I was willing. When I agreed, he asked me to keep him informed about my condition. As soon as I suspected that I might be pregnant again, I let him know and he appeared looking slightly abashed. The good Pandit took an ordinary dropper and ever so carefully tipped into my right nostril two drops of the juice extracted from new shoots of banyan leaves. This went on for four days and I valiantly stifled my giggles and the strong urge to sneeze, for my mentor assured me that because of this treatment, my third child would be a male. In the beginning I scoffed at this idea: "Sex," I said, "is determined at conception." Even *zenana* women knew that! But ayurvedic medicine does not agree.

I remember doubting my own convictions as more than seven months later, I watched the midwife cut my son's umbilical cord! Cord cutting is a moving ceremony with Rajputs, like it is with most other Hindus. It is one of the *sanskars*, the rites of progress in life, and it is done with a ceremonial sword. Only a few hours thereafter, the child's father performs the next *sanskar*, the *jatkarma* or *garhuti*, when he takes a gold coin, dips it in a mixture of honey and clarified butter, and puts a few drops in the little one's mouth.

The palace greeted my son's birth with unprecedented jubilation. But my husband had been just as pleased with his daughters as he then was with his son. I remember him murmuring his blessing to my newborn daughters as he placed the coin on their lips: "may you be as pure as the river Ganga, as wise as Saraswati, the goddess of wisdom, as ideal a woman as Sita."

Had Jijabai been there she might have added under her breath, "and may your body be quite hairless." Women in India have a fixation about body hair—there must be none anywhere, except of course, splendid hair on the head. All three of my children were subjected to hair removing treatment almost the moment they were born. As soon as they emerged and the cord was cut, their little bodies were rubbed everywhere with the placenta. This is a custom in Maharashtra, where Jijabai came from; and I have seen that it really works.

ther women have told me of slight variations, such as rubbing the newborn with blood squeezed from the severed umbilical cord, or with white of egg, kept ready in the delivery room especially for this purpose. But the fact remains that it does work. My daughters, like Jijabai, never had any body hair. In parts of India where this treatment is not practiced, other hair removal methods are used as the children grow up because almost everywhere people are very sensitive of hair on arms, legs, in the pubic areas, and on the face. They would rather that the skin be smooth and hairless.

That is something Miss Blake always found very strange; but I pointed out that English people have such fair body hair that they never have to worry about it. Our hair is darker, so Indian mothers or their nannies spend hours rubbing babies and small children with various ingredients which really do leave the skin hairless.

One of my husband's cousins, who is from central India, told me that when she was a baby, her maids rubbed her all over with a dough made of husked black lentils, ground together with chickpea flour, a teaspoon of turmeric powder, and little bit of water. Where she grew up this was done to

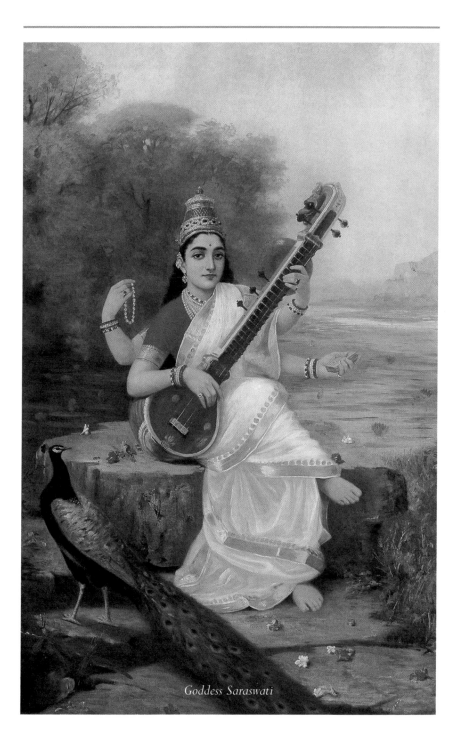

Goddess Saraswati

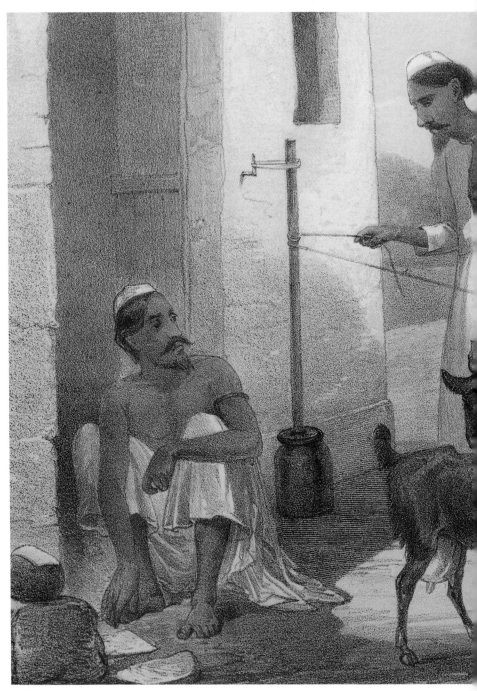

Milking goats

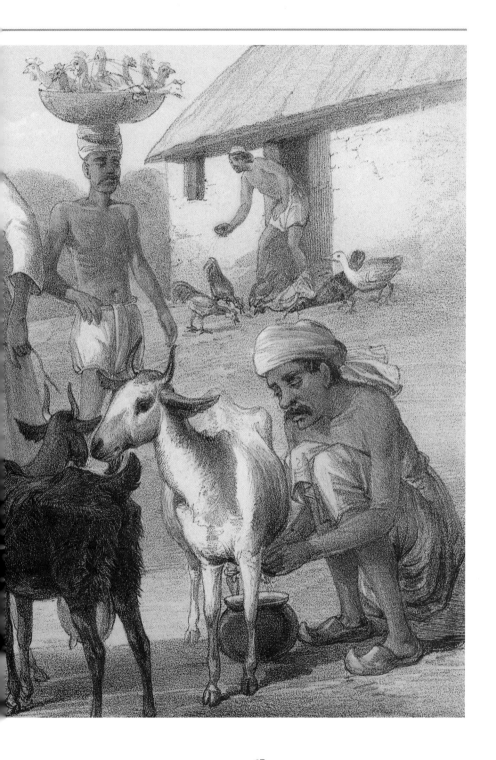

babies for at least six months; "Even to boys" she laughed, "so they wouldn't look like great hairy bears!" This treatment for boys is less common, but most people are convinced it must be done to girls and while they are young. After a certain age, it is no longer effective. In the north, they use dough made of wheat flour and turmeric rather than the husked black lentils. Elsewhere they use egg white, but this is expensive. Whatever the ingredients, they are rubbed on the child's body, allowed to dry completely, then removed by stiff rubbing with a little oil in the palms of the hands.

Dai-Ma used to combine this hair removal procedure with the children's daily massage. Because they had already undergone the placenta rubbing at birth, she merely followed through that treatment with a daily rubbing of goat's milk, which she claimed removed any recalcitrant hairs and left the skin extremely soft. Goat's milk was a favorite of hers, because goats, unlike cows or buffaloes, will only eat fresh greens and therefore their milk is very cooling and pure. I guess Mahatma Gandhi agreed with her, because he too drank only goat's milk.

In any case, Dai-Ma massaged the babies every morning until they were six months old. I loved to watch that procedure, because the babies enjoyed it so much. Dai-Ma would sit on the ground with her legs stretched straight out in front of her; then she'd lay the little one on her legs, right where the calves form a natural well. The babies relaxed completely, smiling into Dai-Ma's eyes when they lay on their backs and resting their little cheeks between her ankles when they were laid on their tummies. They always looked as though they had been made to fit there with their bottoms sticking up in the air!

When I went home for my second confinement my mother advised me to massage my daughter myself. It's a very good postnatal exercise for a new mother, she said. I had watched Dai-Mai oiling my first daughter, so by that time I knew exactly how it should be done.

Dai-Ma would take a bit of oil in her palms and begin a very gentle massage: the legs, chest, arms, and stomach of the child all got a thorough rubbing. She would finish off with the top of the head, the little soft spot, which we call the *taloo*. We believe that rubbing in oil there helps those fontanel bones to grow together, but Miss Blake used to write and say, "Please don't do this." Perhaps the English think it's very dangerous.

But as far as I know, it's done everywhere here. In Kashmir and the north of India, clarified butter is used instead of oil: they actually soak a bit of cotton wool in clarified butter and leave this on the soft spot for fifteen or twenty minutes while they do the massage. The way Dai-Ma did it, there was more to the massage than just rubbing in oil.

he would take their little limbs and gently exercise them, pulling and stretching them in a way that always made them laugh with the sweet toothless smile of that age. She would spend a lot of time gently rubbing and pulling the toes and fingers, to "shape" them. Then she'd do something which amused Miss Blake to no end when I wrote to her about it. Dai-Ma would dip her finger in glycerine, put it into the baby's mouth and gently press up on its palate, the object being to push up the little nose, so it would have a nice shape when the child grew bigger. That reminded me of my own childhood. I remembered that until I was almost five or six, my massage woman would rub the bones of my nose from the outside, pressing up and down, up and down, while she murmured to me, "Did a buffalo step on your nose little one? I'd better shape it, pull it up a bit or how shall we find you a husband?" Somehow I never liked her to do that to me, and yet I allowed the same treatment for my children. I suppose it's hard to break with tradition.

There was another tradition that used to frighten me, but Dai-Ma said we must do it. It is called *galo karna*, and involved pressing the child's throat very gently on the portion where the tonsils grow inside. She would massage this area with an up and down motion, assuring me that this would prevent tonsillitis. I could not protest, because she seemed to be right. At least, none of my little ones suffered from it. We have a saying that "health is worth a thousand other gifts," and I suppose it is to ensure the child's health and sound body from its earliest days that we do all these strange things and

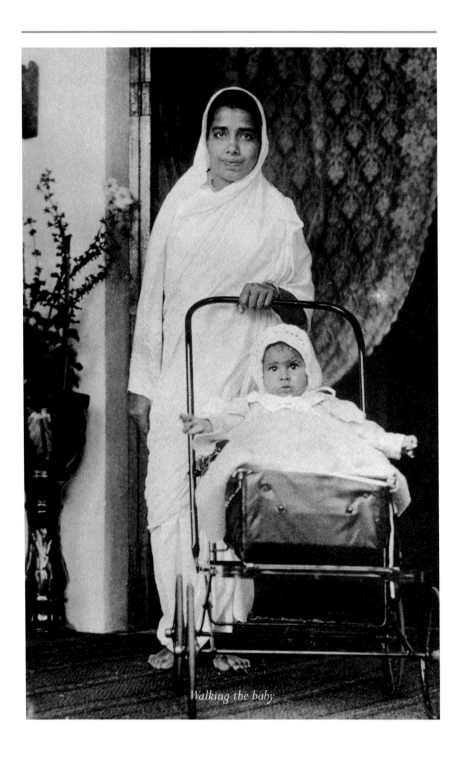

Walking the baby

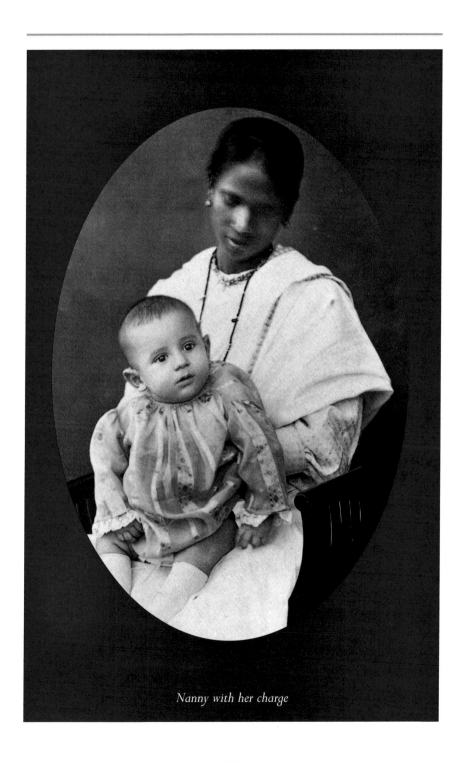

Nanny with her charge

perform so many ceremonies. In the first months of their lives there would be several such ceremonies.

On the sixth and tenth days of the baby's life there are more purification rites and then there is the *namkaran* ceremony of naming the child. Among many Rajputs, this takes place on the twelfth day for a boy and thirteenth for a girl. I used to watch it and think how pretty and colorful the lacquer-work *jhoola* cradles were, in which the baby was swung during the ceremony. For the occasion, the cradles were beautifully decorated with garlands of fragrant flowers. In many parts of India, women choose to keep their babies in a *godhia*, which is a baby-sized hammock, deep and soft. Hung from a rafter, it holds the child quite snugly, just like a womb. Folds of cotton wool or fabric are kept on either side of the baby's head so that the head does not flatten and get misshapen.

raditionally in Rajasthan, it is a paternal aunt who places the child in its cradle for the naming ceremony. Five ladies of the child's clan then swing the cradle gently, singing traditional cradle songs. The same aunt who places the child in the cradle then puts the mark of red *kumkum* powder on its forehead. Then she or the child's mother whispers the chosen name in its ear. The name is then pronounced before the guests and the family gods and sweets are distributed. I used to love this ceremony.

In many places it is also the occasion for piercing the child's ears, and in the case of a girl, for piercing her nose through one nostril as well. In Madanpur, as elsewhere, this was done by the goldsmith. I remember a verse in the medical text, *Sushruta Samhita*, which I read with Pandit Dubey. It states that "the lobules of the ear of an infant are usually pierced through for protecting it from evil influences of malignant stars and spirits and for purposes of ornamentation."

Sushruta wrote that treatise almost two thousand years ago, but ear piercing for protection is still practiced in the country today. My grandmother used to tell me that the women of her generation hardly ever suffered from asthma or other respiratory ailments. They had their ears pierced in the four or five different points where the nerves that affect these ailments are supposed to be located. Today, of course, this is the science of acupuncture. They also wore earrings made of special metals prescribed by their pandits to counteract respiratory complaints.

I have seen in North India how professional ear piercers called *bindanwallas* went from lane to lane shouting, "*Kaan banwa lo*" (get your ears pierced). They usually appeared after the month of March when the warm weather began. Unlike other parts of India where thin gold wires are put in the newly pierced ears, in North India these men used little zinc rings and, believe it or not, some women rubbed rat droppings on their lobes to heal the new aperture!

I never did such things to my children. They all had their ears pierced by the goldsmith, but without the benefit of rat droppings! When the goldsmith came to do his piercing, all the ladies of the family would be present to give their opinions. He would first decide exactly which points he wanted to pierce and then mark them with a dot of saffron. The ladies would nod their approval solemnly if the dots were perfectly placed on both earlobes. The goldsmith would then pierce in exactly the manner prescribed by Sushruta so many centuries ago. "Having soothed the infant and lured it with playthings, the physician should draw down with his left hand the lobules of the child's ears with a view to detect by natural sunlight the closed apertures that are naturally found to exist in these localities. Then he should pierce them straight through with a needle held in his right hand."

The text goes on to say that "plugs of cotton lint should be inserted into the holes of the pricked lobules and lubricated with any unboiled oil." Many people mix a little turmeric with this oil to hasten the healing. Turmeric seems to crop up everywhere in Indian remedies for all sorts of uses. When the children were growing up we really depended on it. I remember Dai-Ma always kept a little bag, called an *ajibai-cha-batua*, "grandmother's pouch." It was our much-used home remedy kit. Everything in it came from the *pansari,* our local grocer who doubled as a druggist.

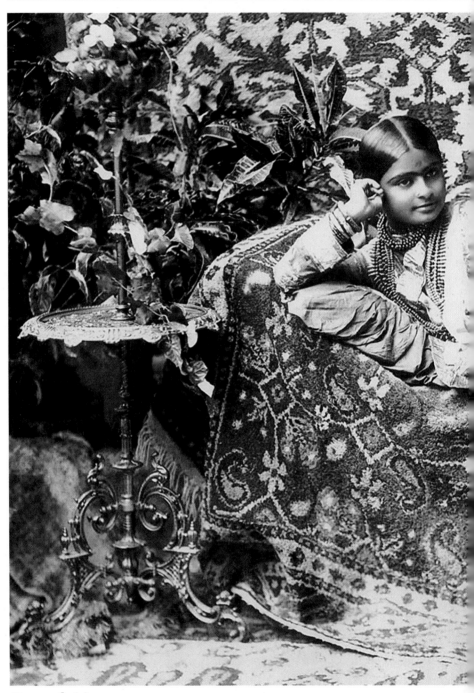

Dreams of adolescence

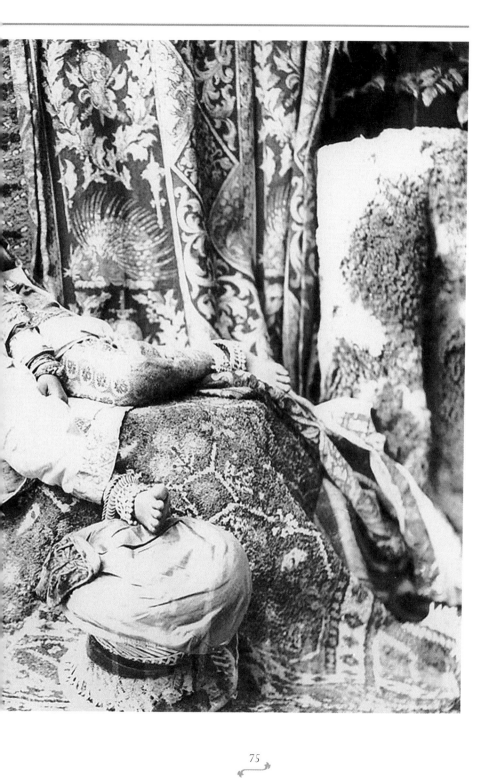

Grandmother's pouch contained about twenty-five herbs, roots, and spices including nutmeg, licorice, long pepper, saffron, sweetflag, bishop's weed, dried ginger, and pomegranate skin. Each ingredient had its own medicinal properties and Dai-Ma knew exactly how many times to rub each ingredient on the special rubbing stone in order to extract just the right strength juice for the treatment. She taught me that these ingredients must always be rubbed clockwise on the stone and for a specified number of rounds, which varied according to the properties of the ingredients and the child's age, with a little water or milk.

All those ingredients were collectively called *bal-gooti*. Of course, there was also turmeric in the pouch. We ran for turmeric rather often as it has beneficial antiseptic and healing properties. I remember once a maid in the *zenana* tripped and cut her chin badly. She refused to go to the doctor, though I was sure she would need stitches. So I sent for the turmeric, scooped out a big spoonful and pressed it against the wound on her chin. The flesh was literally hanging from the wound, so I held it as best as I could with a bandage. Believe it or not, when I opened the bandage two days later, the wound had filled up, and ultimately healed with hardly any scar.

I was impressed, but my doubting husband could not believe his eyes when I showed him. He always teased me about taking my remedies too seriously. I know there's danger of taking too much in your own hands when it comes to health problems. "A little knowledge is a dangerous thing," Miss Blake used to say. We say the same thing a bit differently: "Look at that silly mouse," goes the proverb. "He's found a little piece of turmeric and he is so vain, he's set up his own druggist shop!" The meaning is the same, but I still feel that turmeric never hurt anyone, and there is no doubt it can help.

I used to give turmeric to the children as an alternative to basil-leaf tea. I mixed it with sugar in a cup of hot milk, whenever they suffered from a cough or cold. Just half a teaspoon was enough. In South India, they mix it with a powder of husked green gram and make a paste that they rub on their children like soap. This cleans the skin, protects it from infection, and absorbs any traces of the sesame oil with which the children are massaged.

They also use fresh turmeric rhizome, not the dry powder, on girls reaching puberty to remove hair from the upper lip, sideburns, and forehead.

As much as Indians dislike body hair, we are very proud of the hair on our heads. Still, the hair on the head of the newborn baby is considered unclean and is removed. Among those of the Muslim religion, this removal is not exactly a religious ceremony, it is more of a custom based on the belief that the *jamaal baal*, or birth hair, is unhygienic. Usually the baby's uncle recites a *bismillah*, a small prayer for protection, and holds the child in his lap while the barber shaves the little head quite bald. Sometimes a live goat is killed after this ceremony. Its meat is distributed to family members and to the poor in memory of the first haircut.

or Hindus, the cutting of the first baby hair is another of the sixteen *sanskars*. Before the hair removal ceremony come three other important *sanskars*: first, *nishkraman*, when an auspicious day is chosen and the baby is taken out of the house for the first time; second, *suryavalokan*, when the child is put outside for the first time to worship the sun; and third, *annaprashan*, when the baby eats his first solid food.

The hair removal *sanskar* is called *mundan* or *choodakarma*. It is usually performed when the bones of the soft spot have grown together. Both Muslim and Hindus believe that this first hair must never be trampled on. For that reason it is usually tied in a packet and immersed in some form of moving water. Indians would consider it most inauspicious to save a little piece of hair and keep it in a book as Miss Blake did with her daughter's first chestnut locks.

All these customs and beliefs vary so much even within India. For example, the priestly Brahmin community of Maharashtra, where my massage woman came from, perform the ceremony only for their sons at the age of three years. They never cut a daughter's hair at all. During *mundan*, orthodox Hindus perform many of the ceremonies associated with weddings. These include lighting the sacred fire and rubbing the child's body and head with sweet-smelling preparations of various essences and herbs.

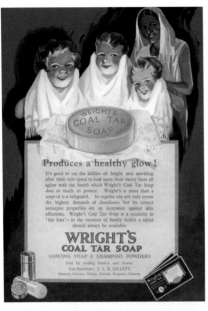

Produces a healthy glow!

It's good to see the kiddies all bright and sparkling after their rub—good to look upon their merry faces all aglow with the health which Wright's Coal Tar Soap does so much to protect. Wright's is more than a soap—it is a safeguard. Its regular use not only serves the highest demands of cleanliness but its correct antiseptic properties are an insurance against skin affections. Wright's Coal Tar Soap is a necessity in 'the East'—in the interests of family health a tablet should always be available.

WRIGHT'S
COAL TAR SOAP
SHAVING SOAP & SHAMPOO POWDERS

Sold by leading Dealers and Stores.
Sole Distributor: T. S. R. GILLETT,
Bombay, Calcutta, Madras, Karachi, Rangoon, Colombo.

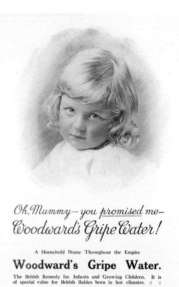

Oh, Mummy — you promised me —
Woodward's Gripe Water!

A Household Name Throughout the Empire

Woodward's Gripe Water.

The British Remedy for Infants and Growing Children. It is of special value for British Babies born in hot climates. ∷ ∷

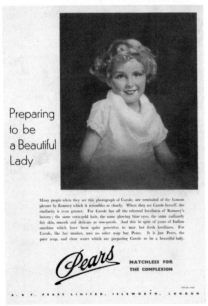

Preparing to be a Beautiful Lady

Many people when they see this photograph of Carole, are reminded of the famous picture by Romney which it resembles so closely. When they see Carole herself, the similarity is even greater. For Carole has all the ethereal loveliness of Romney's beauty; the same corn-gold hair, the same glowing blue eyes, the same radiantly fair skin, smooth and delicate as rose-petals. And this in spite of years of Indian sunshine which have been quite powerless to mar her fresh loveliness. For Carole, like her mother, uses no other soap but Pears. It is just Pears, the pure soap, and clear water which are preparing Carole to be a beautiful lady.

Pears

MATCHLESS FOR
THE COMPLEXION

A. & F. PEARS LIMITED, ISLEWORTH, LONDON

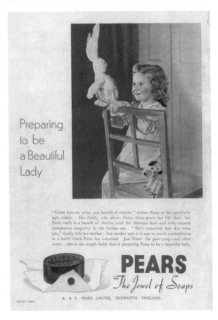

Preparing to be a Beautiful Lady

"Come into my arms, you bundle of charm," recites Patsy to her peculiarly ugly rabbit. Her daddy, who adores Patsy, often greets her like that; but Patsy really is a bundle of charm, with her chestnut hair and rosy-smooth complexion unspoiled by the Indian sun. "She's inherited that skin from you," daddy tells her mother; but mother says it is not so much a complexion as a habit which Patsy has inherited. Just Pears—the pure soap—and clear water...this is the simple habit that is preparing Patsy to be a beautiful lady.

PEARS
The Jewel of Soaps

A. & F. PEARS LIMITED, ISLEWORTH, ENGLAND.

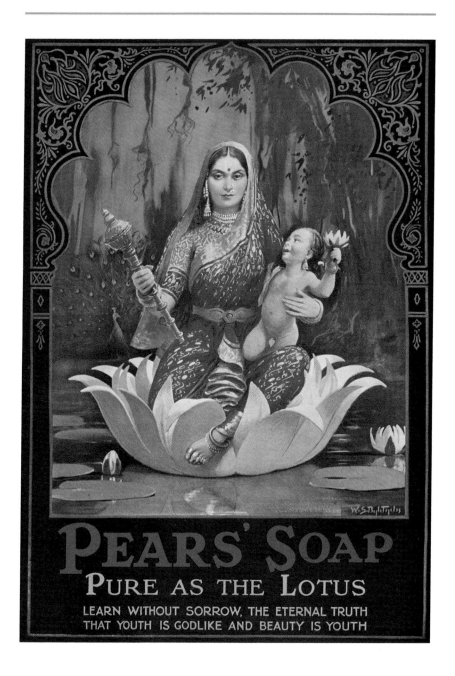

PEARS' SOAP
PURE AS THE LOTUS
LEARN WITHOUT SORROW, THE ETERNAL TRUTH
THAT YOUTH IS GODLIKE AND BEAUTY IS YOUTH

I never used to put any fragrant essences on my babies; I loved their sweet, natural smell. In fact, when they were tiny, we did everything possible to treat them softly and very gently. I remember their little square wooden combs with teeth on both sides, which we used to get from Bengal; they were so gentle on the scalp. Then my mother had taught me the trick of blowing lightly on babies' fingernails to soften them so the nails peel off easily; no need for scissors. I was always afraid of scissors, even the ones made especially for babies that Miss Blake sent me from England.

Eyes are another sensitive area. I used to use a very diluted solution of pure rose water to keep the little ones' eyes clean and free from infection. My husband's grandmother told me that village women, who don't have such nice things as rose water, sometimes put a few drops of their own breast milk into the child's eyes to keep them free from infection and what could be handier! They also put *kaajal* all around the child's eyes to protect them; big black smudges of lampblack, as Miss Blake called it. She thought it looked messy and awful even though I tried to explain that *kaajal* is good for the eyes because it's made of such beneficial ingredients. *Kaajal* is really oily soot. It is gathered in a little container and turned over a flame. Various ingredients burn in this flame, yielding their goodness to the soot. There must be dozens of different recipes for making *kaajal* in India, but I have always made the one my mother taught me; it is excellent and it doesn't seem to smear. I believe this recipe originally comes from Kashmir. It's rather tedious to describe, but so many people ask me that I think I shall record it anyway.

A few days before you are going to make the *kajaal*, take a clean glass vessel and prepare in it a solution of 100 ml (3 ½ cups) of rose water and 5 grams (1 teaspoon) of *rasanjan*. *Rasanjan* is an extract from the stem and root of the *daru-halad* plant, *Berberis aristata* in Latin, commonly called barberry. According to Pandit Dubey, this *rasanjan* was used even by the ancient Greeks to cure opthalmic disorders. Keep stirring this solution for a few days until it is thoroughly mixed, then strain it. At that point it can be used all by itself to clear up infection, a few drops a day in the eyes.

But if you wish to make *kaajal*, then mix this solution with 2 teaspoons of freshly ground turmeric powder, 2 ground almonds, and 2 *nimbu* or lime leaves which have been dried and powdered. Prepare a thick flat roll of cotton wool, like a wick, and soak it in the mixture. Let the wick dry and then twist it tightly. Place it in a little flameproof cup, preferably silver, filled with mustard oil or clarified butter. Invert a second little silver or earthenware cup over the wick. Balance it on something so that it rests about an inch from the flame which will now burn as you light the wick in the first cup. You will have to remove the upper cup two or three times and scrape the accumulated soot into a container—we always used pretty little silver boxes. As homemade *kaajal* is made in large batches, you will have to keep adding oil to the bottom of the cup until you have as much *kaajal* as you want.

When it is ready and all safely tucked away in the prettiest box you can find, add as much clarified butter as is necessary to bring the *kaajal* to the consistency of very thick dough. Try to use a silver box for storing, as silver is very cooling to the eyes and the *kaajal* will take on that cooling quality. The whole idea of *kaajal* is that it soothes, cleanses, and protects the eyes, both from infection and from our old obsession, the evil eye.

As I have said, Indians are ever on the alert to ward off this eye. That's why mothers put such big rings of *kaajal* round their children's eyes: to frighten it off. That is also why they will always put a little black dot called a *teet* on a young child's forehead or cheek. It looks something like what Miss Blake used to call a "beauty mark." Sometimes that little dot is also made of *kaajal*; sometimes it is made of what we call "drumsticks," a long podlike vegetable that hangs from a tree. We dry this vegetable, powder it after it blackens, and mix it with water to make that little spot.

But the nicest *teet* is made of tiny white flowers with orange stems called *parijatak* flowers. These lovely, delicate flowers used to fall like a carpet in our garden in the mornings. We soaked their petals for three days in an iron container, then boiled them to make a thick dark paste. *Teet* made from this paste has the beautiful fragrance of the *parijatak* flower in the mornings, while the dew is still on them.

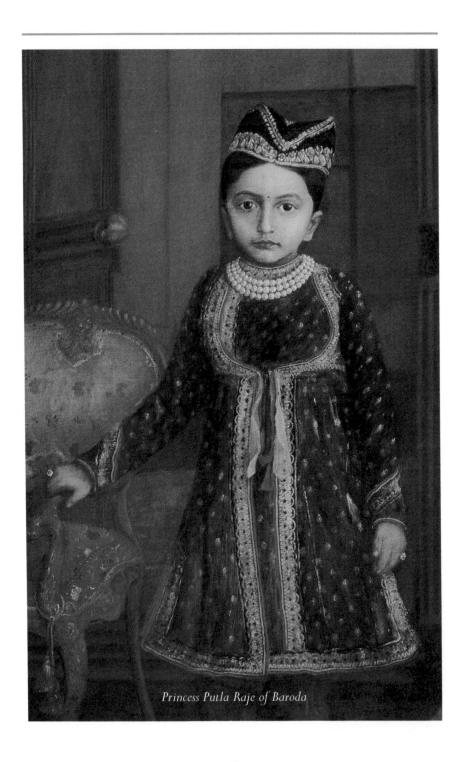

Princess Putla Raje of Baroda

As you can see, avoiding the evil eye is a very complicated business. Piercing the ears and applying *kaajal* and *teet* were some of the ways we did this. Then, of course, there was jewelry. But as far as jewelry for children was concerned, there was more to our theories than just avoiding the evil eye. We also believe that the beneficial qualities of certain metals are actually absorbed into the body through constant contact with the skin. That is why we try to keep a gold or silver chain somewhere on the child's body. Those who cannot afford this thread a metal plaque through black twine and tie that on the hips. There are many people—particularly in villages—who believe such chains prevent hernia.

I put a small gold chain on all of my children. It looked so sweet, I couldn't resist. I also put *walas* on their little feet. *Walas* are anklets made of copper and silver. In those days we put them on to strengthen the child's legs for the first steps. Later, as the child began to walk more surely, we would increase the weight of the anklets. This helps the child to steady her gait, strengthen and balance her step. I might add that the girls' anklets had little silver bells. Their tinkling was a great help in locating them when that steady gait took them out of our sight!

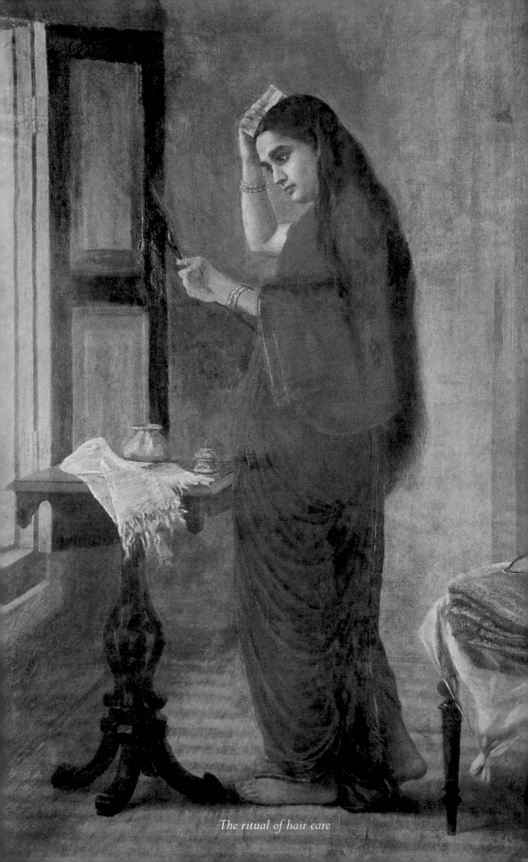

The ritual of hair care

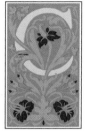 rowning Glory

When the first little pair of feet to wear those tiny anklets were still safely tucked in my tummy, I began to notice, through the haze of happiness at finally becoming pregnant, that my hair was falling out! All my life I had counted on my long, thick black hair to compensate for a face that even my mother consoled me about. I really was rather vain about my hair, so I was desperate to keep it all.

Jijabai came to the rescue. She was a permanent institution in the palace so she was already with me before the baby was born. Her solution was hibiscus oil. She began to rub it into my scalp every morning, explaining that in her part of India, Maharashtra, everyone knew this remedy. The flower is dried and powdered and then mixed with coconut oil. Mind you, only the red hibiscus will do; the other colors are apparently not as effective.

Indian women are very proud of their hair, but to look after it is a pain! Actually, it's a sort of pleasant torture, especially when you are young and impatient to play or do anything but sit still and be oiled, scrubbed, dried, and plaited.

"Hair is an adornment; hair is a plague!" I don't know where that proverb comes from, but it's so true. The whole hair procedure can take hours, and what's more, it cannot be done by one person. Most of the women I've talked to mention one if not two maids or family members helping with the hair ritual. It is no wonder that women of today, especially in cities, are beginning to cut their hair or perm it. They don't have the time or the staff to look after it as we did in the old days.

In those days hair treatment didn't mean a shampoo and set, or a trip to a shop to sit under some sort of machine. It meant lengthy preparation of various oils, decoctions of leaves and herbs, pastes made of things like mud, yogurt, and turmeric, long drying sessions while one's hair was spread out over a smoking basket. All that was for young, healthy hair. When it began to gray, there were still more complicated preparations to make and apply. Yet the results speak for themselves. In my days the norm was knee-length hair, so heavy that sometimes it really was tiring just to balance when it was done up in a bun. But we would never have shorn ourselves like women today. Short hair was only for widows. We tied our hair up in a thousand different, intricate ways; but we left the length as nature intended.

There are many ideas about how to maintain long, clean, healthy hair. When I began to ask my friends, I was surprised at the variety of, for example, falling hair remedies. A friend from Kashmir told me with great conviction that the only thing to do for falling hair was to rub yogurt and mustard oil thoroughly into the scalp. Another lovely woman of sixty-five from Tamil Nadu, whom I met in South India, assured me that for falling hair the only thing was to cut open the bark of a banana tree, remove the sticky substance inside, and rub it into the scalp. I now understand that of course, it all depends on what is readily available and cheap in the place where one lives. In this respect, Mother Nature is so generous in India; she has made provision for everyone's need everywhere.

During my first pregnancy I formed a resolution to learn all that I could about hair. Pandit Dubey's habits must have influenced me because I began to collect and record information like a pandit myself! I even persuaded one of the palace scribes to sit with me and write down information whenever I talked to people. This continued for years, right through my palace days, my travels with my husband, and our brief posting to South India while he was there in the administration. Personal scribes were one of the nice things about being a princess in those days. I shall now indulge myself in sharing a bit of what I recorded while talking with women of my country. For the most part, they shall speak for themselves, because I find each woman's way of speaking has a charm of its own.

I love my South Indian friend's description of how her hair was washed as a child. These are her words telling me of the whole bath routine.

"For the bath ritual we had a special silver vessel with a long silver handle. At the end of it were three little bowls in beautifully chased silver with lovely designs on them. Each one held a different oil: one for the face, one for the body, and one for the hair. Then there was a copper vessel, which held a herbal paste that they used for our hair. That herb was called *thali*, it's a leaf, which they ground fresh every day and the paste it makes is quite thick and green.

"After that shampoo paste was applied, we were bathed in some herbal waters, in which the bark of forty different trees had been boiled. That was *nalpamaravellam*, which means forty-tree-water. It was supposed to be an excellent tonic for the hair, skin, and the body. After the bath, our hair was dried with a thin muslin towel, then spread over a *karandi*, a sort of iron pot with a long handle. In the pot were burning coals with all sorts of herbs sprinkled on them so the smoke became very fragrant. We would dry our hair over this smoke. It was very mild, so the scalp didn't get hot. It also dried the hair very slowly, so the ends never became brittle and it left such a beautiful fragrance. A dry, powdered herb was rubbed in the center of our heads when our hair was dry, only in the middle of the hair parting. That was supposed to prevent colds. The whole thing would take hours. The entire morning would go in this bath. We would get up at six o'clock in the morning, bathe, and go to the temple, come back and have a hot meal which would be served immediately at ten-thirty."

It makes me feel beautiful and indolent, just reading that description. I might add that the lady was a princess of Travancore, now a part of the state of Kerala, and therefore perhaps slightly more indulged than the average South Indian woman. But I think women everywhere spent as much time as they could on their hair, whether they were princesses or not.

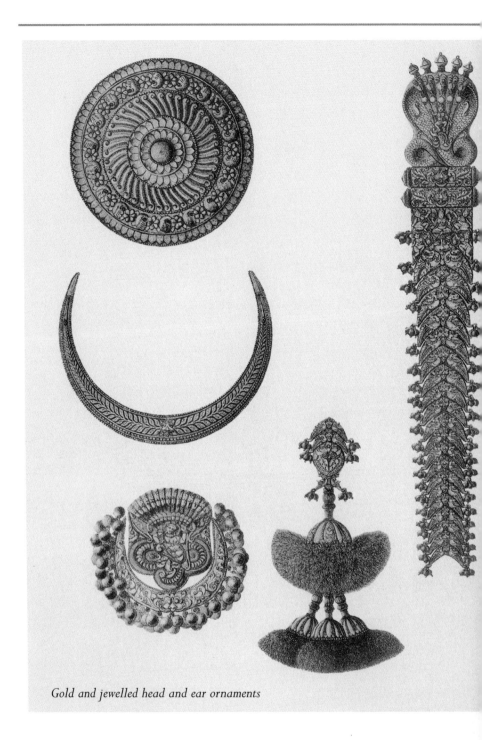

Gold and jewelled head and ear ornaments

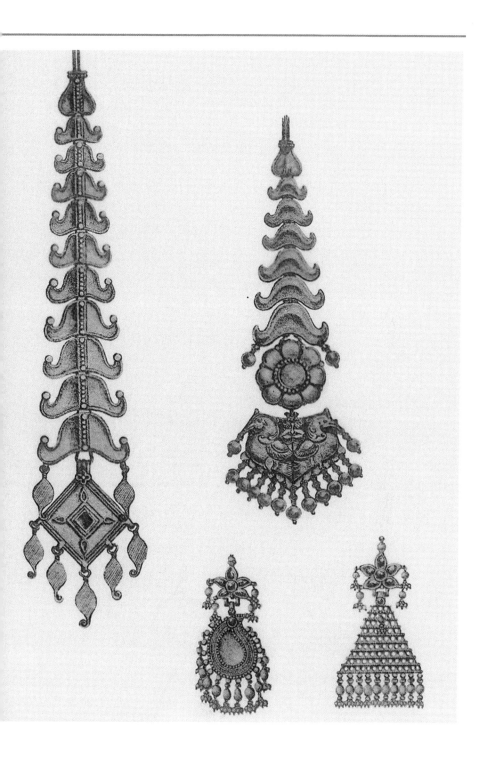

Another friend of mine was from a very good family of Hyderabad, but she was not a princess. She was a Muslim, like the Nizam, Hyderabad's famous ruler, who was once considered the wealthiest man in the world! Muslim traditions are often different from Hindu traditions even though they may coexist in the same region. In this description of her hair care, she also talks about her childhood fifty years ago.

"Of course the biggest ritual was the hair wash; for that they used to oil the hair the night before. In Hyderabad we used *amla* oil, made by extracting the juice of the *amla* fruit and boiling it with pure coconut oil. This oil was rubbed into my scalp the night before the shampoo. Usually it was my mother who did it. She would take a handful of oil, by that I mean a handful, as much as your hand could hold, put it on top of the head and let it soak. Then she or one of the maids would start massaging it. At the end of the massage, there was still a lot left on the top of the head, so the rest of my plait was taken and rubbed in that oil. The hair was never rubbed at the bottom, as I have seen others do; it was only at the scalp; then all the hair was taken on top and tied up in a thin scarf so that the pillow didn't get oily.

"Then they used to boil *shikakai* or *ritha*—also the night before. Sometimes *amla* was added to that. The next day our hair was washed with that solution and again tied up like a turban with muslin cloth. It was sort of wrung out with that cloth. Then they made us lie down. There was a special basket which had fairly big holes—it wasn't a closely woven basket—and this was covered with a pink cloth. Why pink, I don't know. We lay down with our hair spread over this basket and they lit *loban* incense in a little burner called an *ood-daan*. The charcoal was put in this and on it the *loban*; and we had to lie on a rug on the floor till the hair dried. The fragrance lasted a whole week. My mother used to do the same thing. Everything about her smelled of this wonderful herbal incense. She never used perfume. She used the same incense even in her clothes cupboard.

"But I was talking about us girls. When our hair was semi-dry, they used to comb out the knots with an ordinary comb; a brush was never used. Then they would take a few strands of hair from just above the ears and braid it into one thin plait at the back so that the hair stayed out of our faces. You stayed like that till the hair was completely dry. They wouldn't let you braid it even if it was slightly damp because you might catch cold or something. Do you know that the basket for drying our hair was part of our wedding trousseau? It was made very beautifully with bright pink or red satin on it and little gold tassels around each hole.

"Another thing we all loved was flowers. Hyderabad grows beautiful *chameli* and *mogra* jasmine, so every evening all of us girls made a little *veni*, a delicate little garland, which was put through two strands of hair at the top of the plait. We always had flowers in our hair every evening, because it was either *chameli* or *mogra* season. Our hair always smelled of incense and flowers throughout the week."

o there you see what a life people led; so much nicer than beauty parlors! I might explain about *shikakai* and *ritha* because they are quite commonly used for washing hair in various parts of India. *Ritha* is a hard little nut called a soapnut, which you can buy in any provision store. It has to be soaked a long time before you can use it, but when it is softened and boiled in water it makes absolutely natural suds that are good not only for hair but also for washing delicate clothes and jewelry and especially for cleaning pearls!

There is a sister soapnut called the *shikakai* bean, also excellent for shampooing hair. Women all over India have used *shikakai* and *ritha* forever. They have also used *amla* or *aonla* as a conditioner. *Amla* is a sour, astringent fruit (*Phyllanthus embelica* in Latin) which can be dried and boiled with one of the soapnuts as a conditioner, or rubbed fresh onto the scalp to prevent hair loss and dandruff.

Both the Travancore princess and my flower-bedecked friend from Hyderabad cared for their hair with different rituals from those I was accustomed to in Rajasthan. After I married and came to Madanpur, I found that women there used neither *shikakai* nor *ritha* but a pale yellow

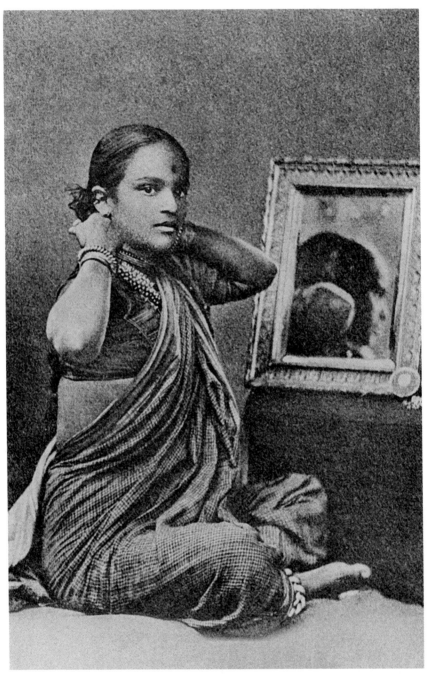

Performing her toilette

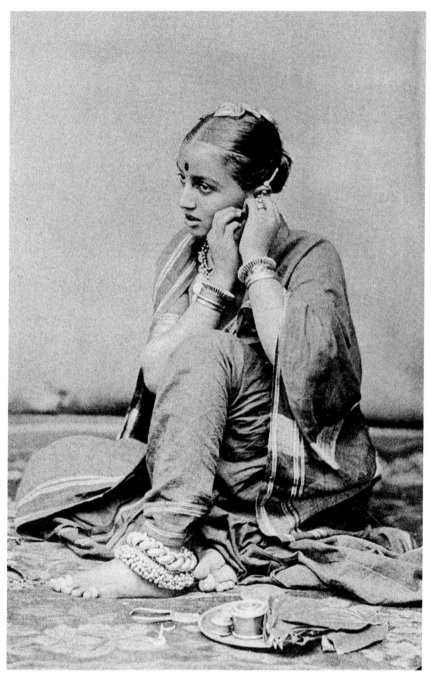

Displaying her ornaments

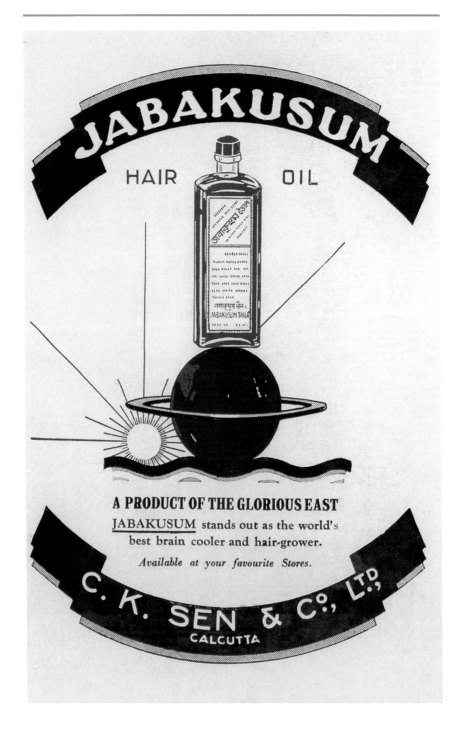

clay called *meth*. That clay was left in water all night; in the morning one of the maids would rub it into a fine paste and add lime juice to it. Sunday was hair-washing day. We used to make a sort of party of it. We all would get together in one of the huge bathing rooms of the *zenana* and scrub that *meth* paste into our hair with the help of the maids. We sat on the silver *bajots*, which were low stools, while they scrubbed and then poured ladles and ladles of hot water over our heads to rinse. The water was kept in big steaming copper cauldrons, as it was commonly believed that copper imparted beneficial qualities to the water.

We would allow ourselves to feel a bit languid and brazen, moving about the bathroom scantily clothed, our hair hanging loose and open. It was a rare indulgence because in public our hair could never be loose. "A woman with her hair down is a harlot," goes the saying. We had always to be smoothly and discreetly coiffed.

In a way, that too had its own satisfaction, but I remember watching the maids in their courtyard, performing their own toilette. I envied them a bit because their hairstyle, called *matha guntho,* was more coquettish than we were allowed, and also much more convenient. They first knotted the hair in the center of the forehead into a gold bead called a *rakhdi*. Then they parted the hair all over the scalp and braided it into the most intricate little plaits which all met at the back to form one big braid. It looked wonderfully neat and tidy and they didn't have to undo their hair for a week. When they did, it was very curly and wavy all the way down, so tempting to touch that I could just look at it and dream of being a languid courtesan.

Of course, there was never a question of anything half so exciting for me! From my earliest days I remember dreaming about how I would grow up to be a modest, devoted wife, the ideal and virtuous Padmini! Such dreams helped to pass the time during tiresome chores like having my long, black hair oiled and combed. "Long black hair, Mother makes it grow. Father buys colored tassels to adorn it." That's the song my mother used to sing while she oiled and combed (but never brushed).

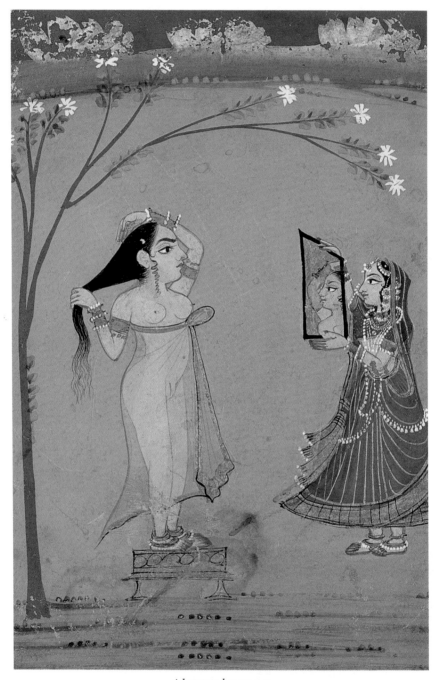

Admiring her tresses

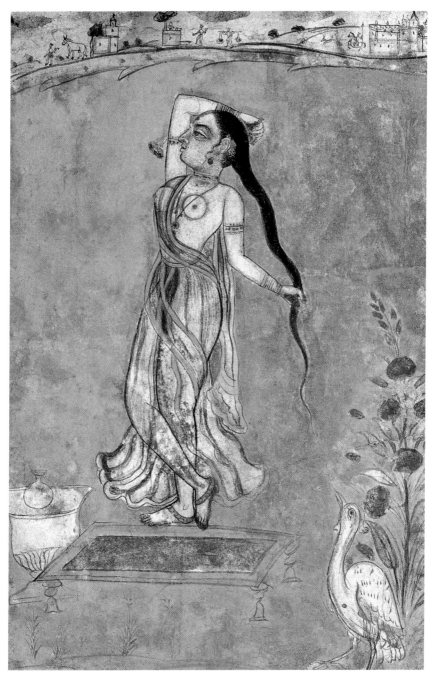

Drying her hair

ntil very recently, Indian women never brushed their hair. We didn't even have brushes traditionally; they were first brought here by Europeans. But we had a wonderful variety of combs: plain ones in ivory, bone, horn, and tortoise shell; and two-pronged ones, like forks for lifting the hair. Some were beautifully designed in brass, silver, and gold. My mother's was shaped like a lovely gazelle, its long horns formed the prongs for combing. But the time it took and the amount of oil! Mother didn't use clarified butter or sesame or castor oil or mustard oil or plain coconut oil like other Indian women I've met. She used the oil of a long marrow squash called *doodhi* that took hours to prepare.

First she collected all the ingredients that her ayurvedic doctor had prescribed. There were leaves of the *brahmi* plant, *jatamansi* (or spikenard), *amla,* and many others. All these herbs and roots were soaked in coconut oil for a day or two until the oil became green. Then mother would grate the marrow into this oil and put the whole thing to cook on the fire. When the marrow was cooked, the oil was strained and bottled. My mother would supervise this work at our New Year, making enough for a full year's supply. She always claimed *doodhi* oil was not only beneficial but also cooling; and I never had reason to doubt her.

I only wished she wouldn't use quite so much. She would part my hair in different places and pour the oil onto the scalp from a silver vessel with a long, thin spout. The massage would start gently at the roots of my hair and would be worked up to a more vigorous rubbing. I knew it was good for me, but I hated it dripping and used to dash off to my father's study as soon as I could to wipe off the excess with his blotting paper.

Miss Blake shared my secret aversion, but she was more vocal about it. "Why do you women drown yourselves in oil like that? A little goes a long way!" I could only quote to her from Pandit Dubey's old *Charak Samhita*: "One who applies oil on his head regularly, does not suffer from headaches, baldness, greying of hair. Nor does his hair fall. The strength

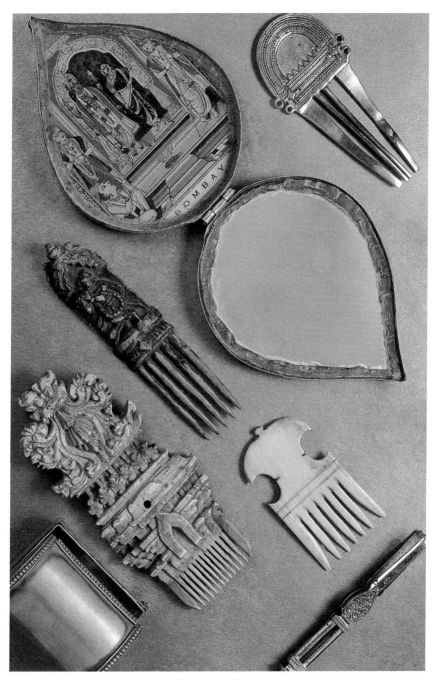

Combs and decorative hair accessories

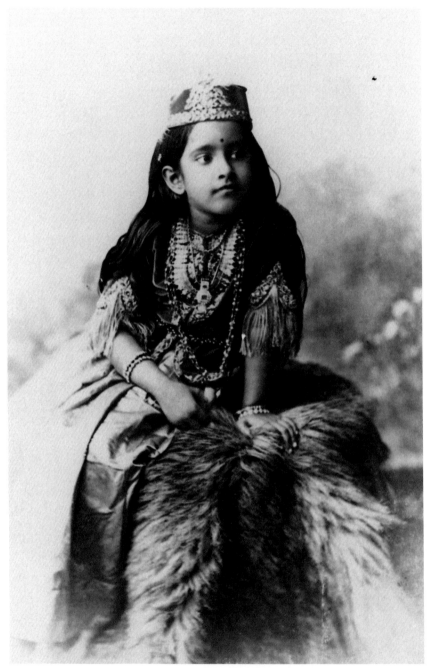

Princess Laxmibai of Travancore

of his head and forehead is specially enhanced; his hair becomes black, long and deep-rooted. His sense organs work effectively. The skin on his face brightens. Applying oil on the head produces sound sleep and happiness."

In the end Miss Blake succumbed ever so slightly and allowed the maids to rub sesame oil on her head ever so often, just for the joy of the massage.

here are many different solutions to the problem of graying. Henna, which we use for staining our hands and feet red, has the same effect on hair, if the hair has become slightly gray. To black hair it will give reddish highlights; gray hair will become red-orange.

Besides henna, the powder of red hibiscus is a remedy for gray hair. Other people use curry leaves, boiled in coconut oil and strained. Still others do the same thing with leaves of the Margosa, the *neem* tree, which are good for so many other things as well. Those are some garden solutions.

The kitchen cupboard also yields lots of possibilities to battle gray. North Indian women often rinse their hair in a strong solution of tea to maintain its color. Others make a decoction of onion seeds that they use as a darkening rinse. In the north where dairy products are available in plenty, women will massage a little cow's milk butter into the hair roots, claiming this arrests the graying process. The same *amla* fruits that are used with *shikakai* as a conditioner can also be used as a dye. Soaking them in an old iron vessel will turn the water purple-black after a few days and it can then be applied very carefully to darken gray hair. But it will also stain the skin, so be careful.

Some people delight in roundabout methods. I have heard several good ones for preparing a hair dye: you can take a little marking nut called *bibba,* boil it in milk, and use that *bibba* milk to fertilize some earth. In that earth, plant fenugreek seeds and when the plants grow, use the leaves to make a hair dye. Alternatively, if you want to make quite a permanent dye, plant fenugreek seeds in the hollow of a "cooling" *neem* tree; pluck the fenugreek leaves from the crevice when they grow, cook them with the *bibba* nut, and use this

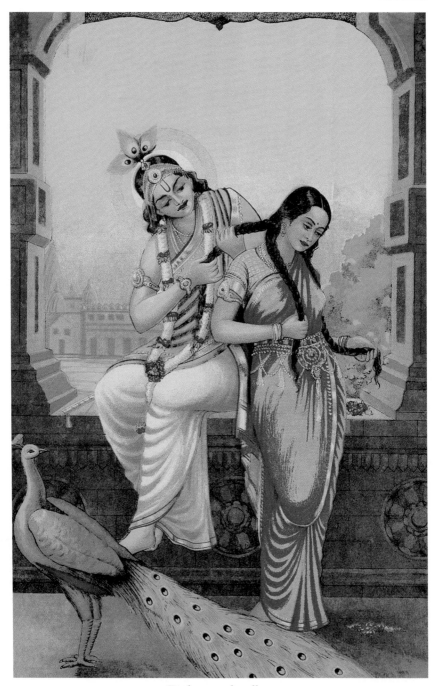

Krishna-venibandhan

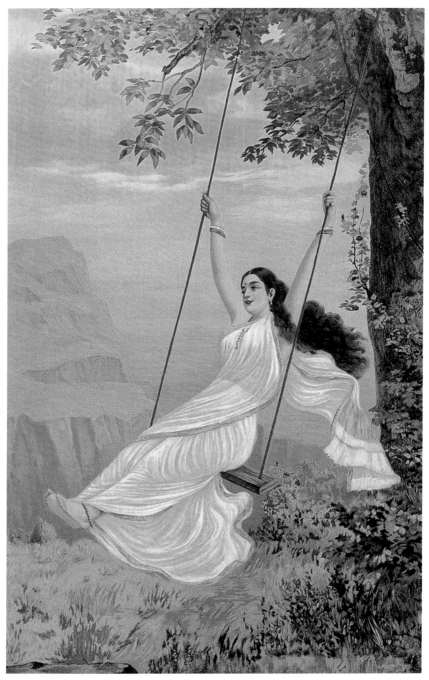

The temptress, Mohini

mixture to darken the hair. People actually did such things once upon a time. Perhaps they still do them somewhere.

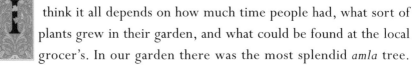I think it all depends on how much time people had, what sort of plants grew in their garden, and what could be found at the local grocer's. In our garden there was the most splendid *amla* tree. Even today it makes my mouth water to think of its fruit. It was so sour and astringent, it made my teeth tingle. How I loved it, fresh from the tree, to nibble with salt and pepper. I suppose none of us knew how rich it was in vitamin C, but my mother surely knew of its other properties. Just as she supervised the making of our hair oil every year, she also oversaw the preparation of our shampoo, which would be made once a week. *Amla* was an essential ingredient. It was soaked overnight with one of the two commonly used soapnuts, *shikakai* or *ritha*, then boiled with one or two herbs and some musk for fragrance, strained and used as our shampoo. The *amla* is essential to soften and condition the hair because soapnuts leave it a little brittle. Some people feel it also prevents dandruff, stimulates hair growth and helps to retard premature graying. You can substitute fresh lemon juice for the *amla* if it is not available.

Amla, in combination with two other common Indian fruits, *bhaira* and *hirada*, makes a mixture called *triphala* "three fruits." *Triphala* can be purchased ready-made at any Indian grocery. It is said to have miraculous medicinal properties for everything from stomach, eye, and teeth ailments to making pickles! Pandit Dubey used to swear by *triphala*, and in particular by the *hirada* fruit (*Terminalia chebula* in Latin). He used to tell us that a regular intake of *hirada* retards the aging process and assures a long and healthy life. He recommended one gram of powdered *hirada* mixed with clarified butter be eaten every day to keep healthy and sharpen the intellect. "When the gods spilt some nectar from the heavens," he would say, "the drops turned into *hiradas!*"

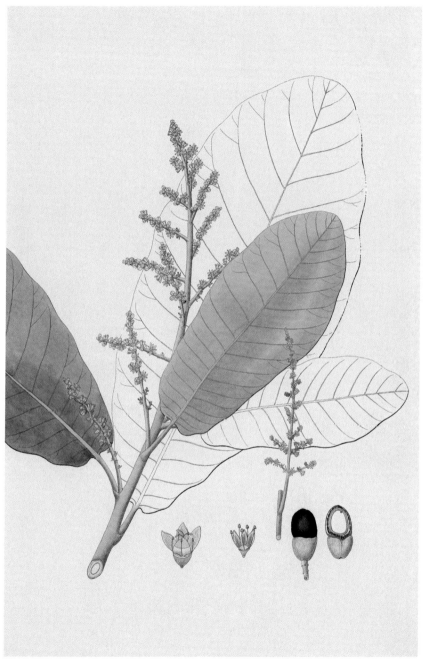

Bibba nut used for dyeing hair.

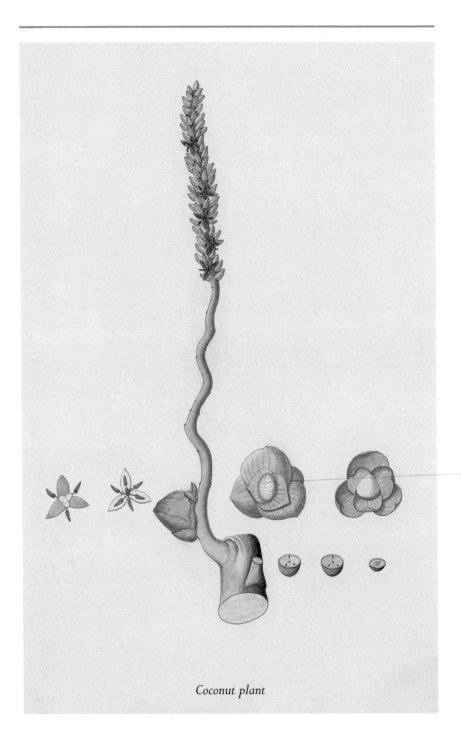

Coconut plant

ut we were talking about hair. Many people suggest using *triphala* as a magic remedy for hair loss and also for conditioning it. Then there are the advocates of *urad dal* or black gram. Soaked overnight and ground into a thick paste, *urad dal* can be massaged into the hair. When it is washed out, it leaves the hair extremely soft. But I cannot imagine how it must feel while that sticky paste is in your hair. The ground leaves of the hibiscus plant, used in many parts of India, are equally sticky, but are said to be excellent for the hair. I cannot imagine also doing as the North Indian women do: dousing my hair with natural yogurt. They swear it is a very effective conditioner, but for me there would be the question of smell. I have heard that women in the western Indian region of Gujarat use buttermilk to wash and condition their hair, but solve the problem of smell by using a little potpourri of fragrant dried herbs known as *khevna*. *Khevna* smoke is good for the hair as well as for clothes that smell musty after the rains.

In areas where there is rice in plenty, women use rice water, strained from their cooked rice, as a simple hair rinse by itself or they mix it with *shikakai* shampoo. Where there are coconuts, women use coconut milk. Jijabai used to tell me of her childhood days in Maharashtra when she and her sisters would take one coconut each, grate them on a grater shaped like the back of a turtle, and squeeze the milk from the grated fruit into the vessel. They would heat that milk slightly, rub it into their hair, and leave it for a short time while they steeped a decoction of fragrant jasmine from their own garden into their *shikakai* shampoo.

I can just imagine them stretched out in the sunlight after the shampoo, their hair spread over a basket of herb incense smoke, lazily watching the parrots in the mango trees and laughing at some silly joke. That sort of vision makes me long to be young again, close to the earth and closer to other women. Somehow in those days we were all sisters in these simple pursuits. That was a very sweet comfort.

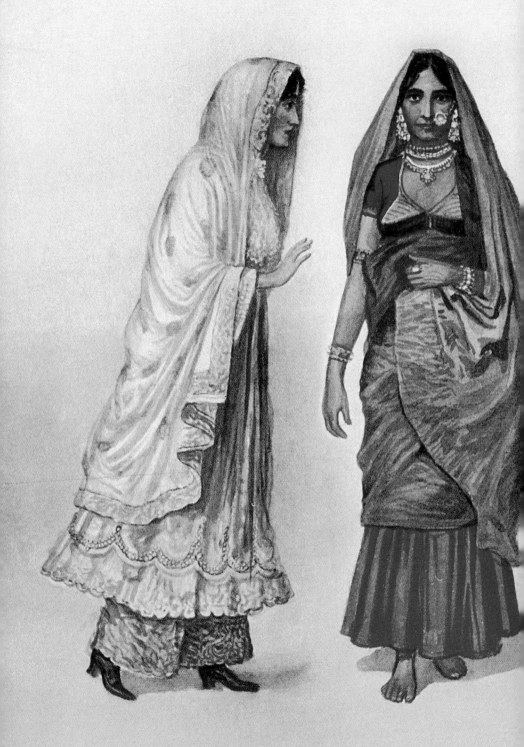

Women of India, watercolors by M. V. Dhurandhar

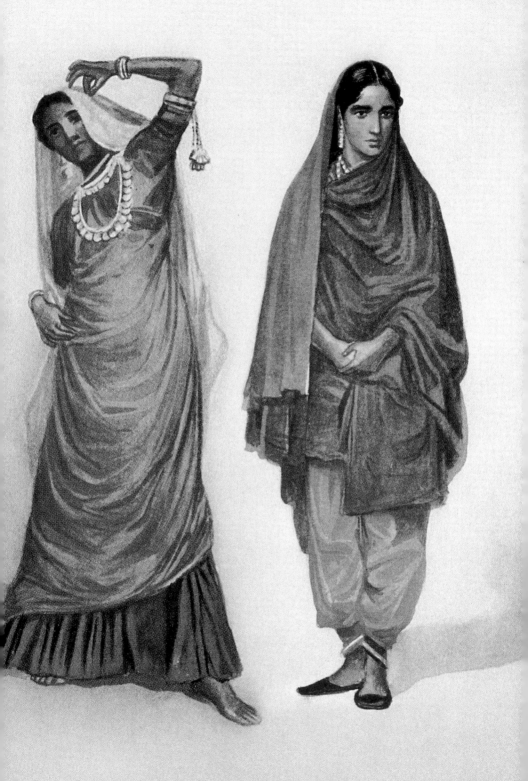

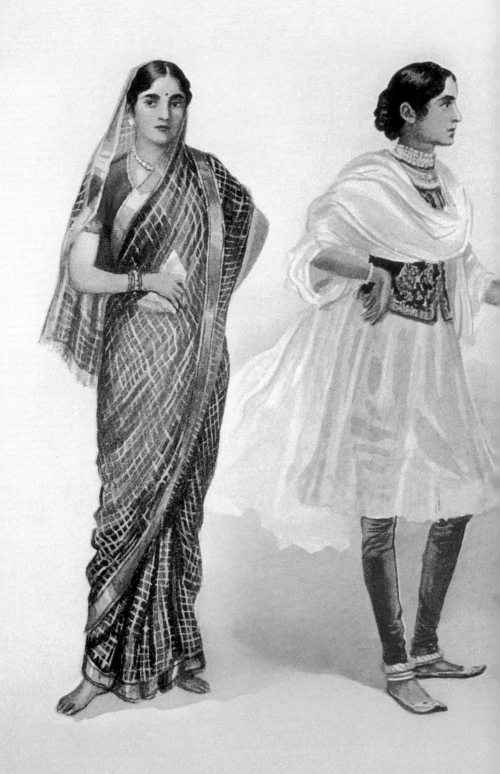

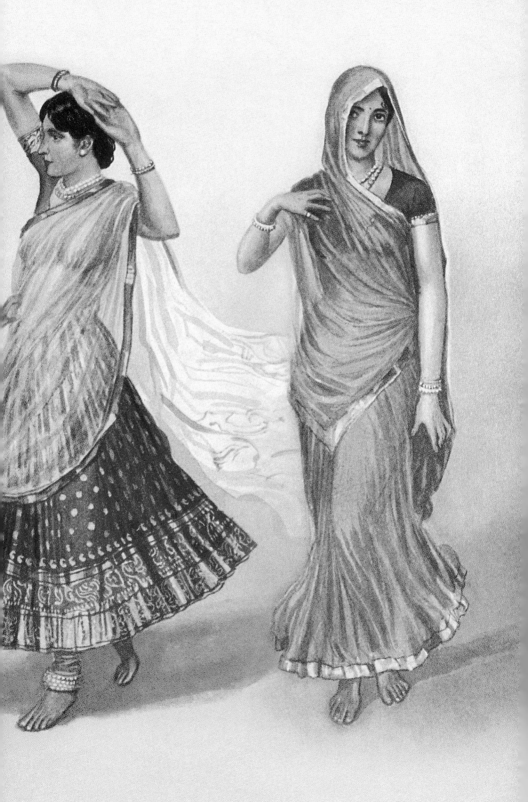

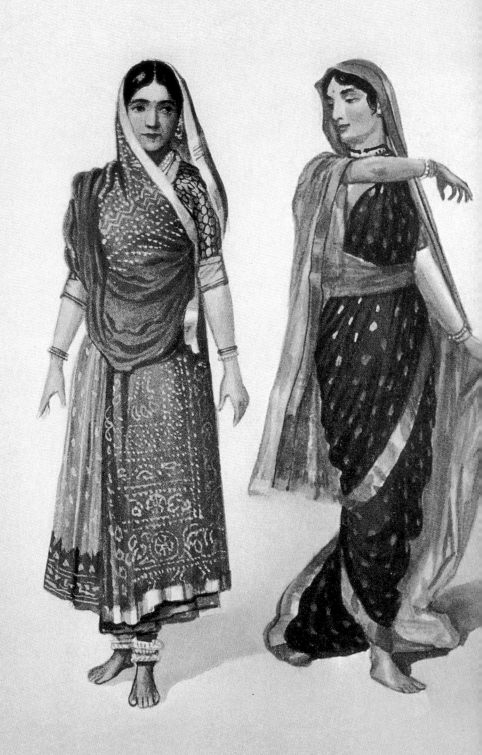

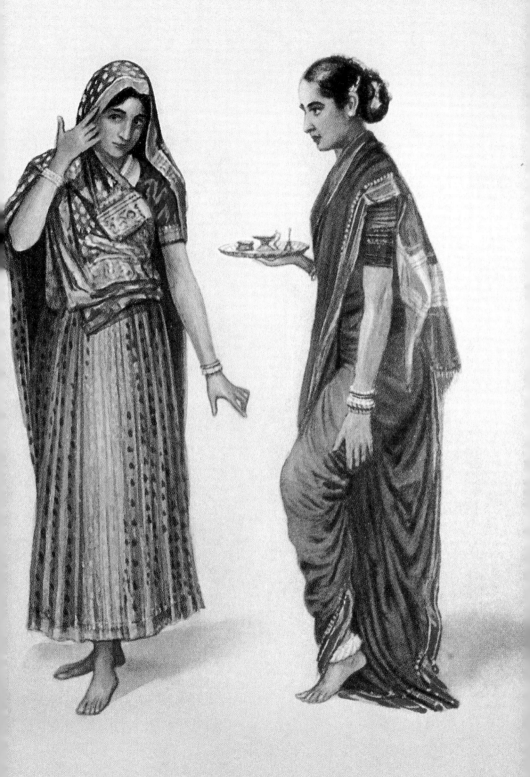

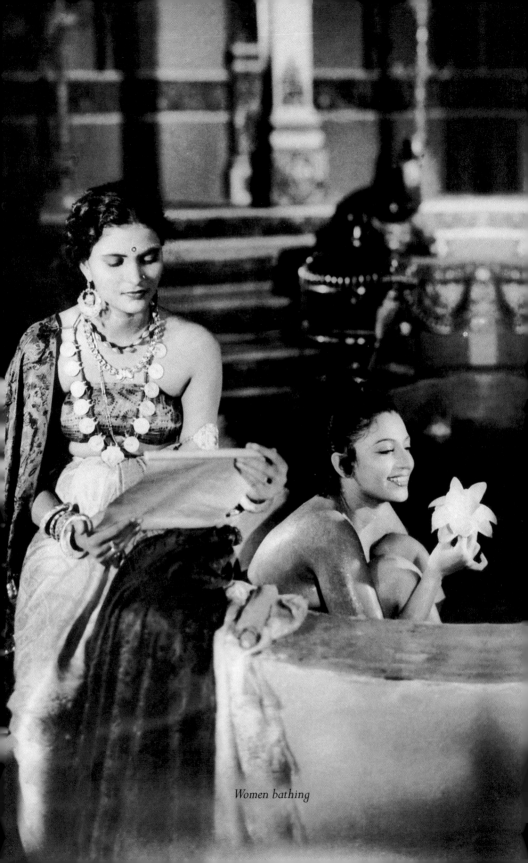

Women bathing

6.

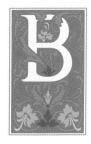athing Beauty

I once went to the cinema in Bombay, long ago, and saw a picture about dolphins playing in the sea. It was full of sunshine and movement and freedom. Those dolphins looked so happy, all sleek in a group; they reminded me of us—we *zenana* women—on a Sunday morning having our bath. I can't remember ever being more relaxed and contented than on those Sunday mornings. The bathing area was our haven.

It was the only place in our regimented world where we could move about barely clothed, our hair open, and our tongues loose. My goodness, I learned a lot while scrubbing and sluicing. I have never felt anywhere else in my life as safe and secure and utterly happy as I did in those old bathing rooms. Every detail of them sticks in my mind as though the objects themselves were old friends.

The bathroom was the size of a palace bedroom and it opened onto a private courtyard. Needless to say, men never set foot anywhere near this area. It was totally our own domain. Outside in the courtyard were the big, old *hamams*, pot-bellied water heaters made of copper, which shone so softly with age and endless polishing. The maids would scrub them every week with ash and tamarind pulp. The water that came out from them was steaming hot and coppery tasting. A fire crackled below and smoke puffed out through old iron chimneys. The *hamam* was a fantastic contraption.

When I was a girl, there was no running water in my father's palace. The maids would carry in steaming cauldrons of water and dump it into big *ghangals*, containers of copper and silver. Being in contact with these metals was supposed to make the water more beneficial.

In the middle of the bathing room was a sort of black stone platform with a rough top, pitted like one of the stones we used for grinding spices in the kitchen. That rough, raised surface kept us from slipping in spite of all the oils and unguents we used during the bath. Being higher than the floor, it proved a dry little island and we dressed on this after the bath. But we also used it like a big foot scrubber. We could rub our heels and the sides of our feet on it and any roughness would disappear. As we were almost always barefooted or in open sandals, our feet tended to get rough more often than Miss Blake's. She always kept her feet securely hidden in big shoes with laces.

In fact, we never saw her feet except in the bath, and even there she seemed more shy of those feet than of any other part of her body. That made us look at them and of course, we too thought they looked a bit defenseless and sort of exposed. Miss Blake's feet were much more fragile than our own. From the time we were babies, we had treated our feet almost like hands. We massaged them with oils and unguents and softened them with ordinary butter or with *kokam* butter. *Kokam* butter is made from a deliciously sour fruit, sometimes called the wild mangosteen, grown on the west coast of India.

We adorned our feet with tinkling anklets, and after marriage with henna and toe-rings. We used our feet in so many ways. They were friendly things, not only for dancing or tickling or wiggling the toes; but also for work. I remember the cook used to hold the handle of his big knife with his toes. The blade stuck straight up in the air with its sharp side away from his body and he cut his meat against it, with both his hands free! There was also the man who used to make lac bangles for us; he held many of his tools with his feet. My maids were forever using their feet for things like making rope for hanging a baby's hammock, twisting the fiber to make twine.

Now such familiar and useful things as feet have to be kept very clean. Most Indians will wash their hands and feet morning and evening, I suppose, even if there is not enough water to douse the whole body. It's like an obsession with us. I remember we used to have lovely little scrubbers, apart from the big stone, for rubbing difficult places on the feet. They were made of brass or copper, the lower side flat, with deep crisscrosses to make them abrasive. The top was a beautifully crafted bird or animal that served as the handle. A friend of mine from Hyderabad told me that a scrubber was part of her trousseau. In her part of India, it was made from a natural porous stone, very much like pumice stone but brick colored. For the trousseau, the stone would be carved into different shapes, and if you could afford it, there would be a decorative silver handle on top. As part of her trousseau, my friend was also given a *chauki*, a little marble stool for sitting and sluicing herself during the bath.

Bathing was always pure pleasure. We have a saying, "You can eat and regret; but not bathe and regret." This passion we all have for bathing probably stems from the climate we live in. Anyone who lives "down country," (anywhere south of Delhi), feels they must bathe at least once a day, and jumps at the chance to bathe more often. "A man's bath and a woman's dinner are soon over," is a proverb which leads me to think that perhaps it is women more than men who really revel in this pursuit and prolong it as much as possible. I know for a fact that many Hindu women in various regions would still never dream of cooking in the morning without first bathing and performing their *puja*, the ritual "good morning" to their gods.

Now with all this talk of bathing, you might imagine, as Miss Blake did at first, that tub makers in India do a booming business. Not at all! In fact, very few people bathe in a tub. Most would prefer to sit or stand next to a vessel full of water and sluice themselves with a mug called a *lota*. We feel this is cleaner and more satisfying than sitting in stagnant water. And we go about that sluicing with gusto!

Oh, poor Miss Blake! At first she found the whole thing extremely off-putting because we even clean the insides of our noses, sniffing in and sneezing out water for all the world like an old elephant. We gargle and spit, we even scrape our tongues using horseshoe-shaped wire, and fiddle about with our ears to remove any hidden dirt or wax. The truth is that in a climate like ours, where there is so much dust and continuous heat, you must do all this to keep healthy.

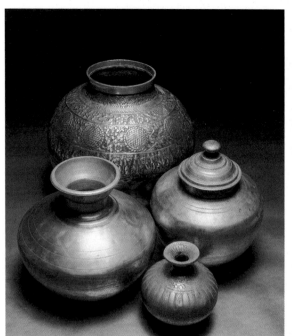

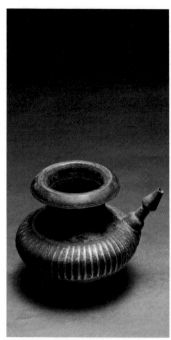

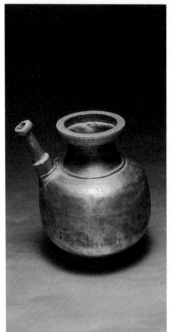

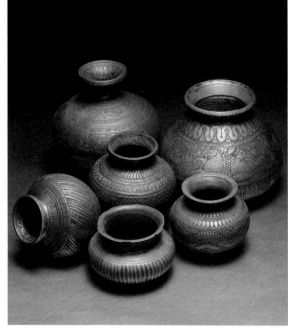

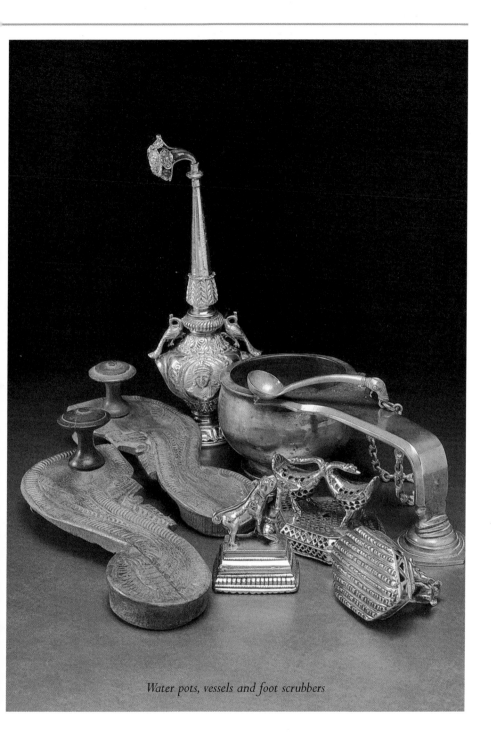

Water pots, vessels and foot scrubbers

In the end Miss Blake understood, and even came to join us in the bathing rooms, believe it or not. After about a year of tubbing in private all alone in her little suite, she asked me one Sunday if we would mind, and I remember trying hard not to smile. It was funny and sweet to watch her with us, gradually relaxing, letting her towel slip and scrubbing herself, as we did, with the special yellow clay called *meth* which we also used for washing our hair. Soap was still not in vogue in that period. We knew about it but we considered it much too drying to the skin. I remember my father actually forbade his women to use soap, especially on our faces.

This clay business was all right as long as our bathing rooms were big and old-fashioned, with plenty of maids to scrub them. But I remember my aunt telling us about the senior maharani of a neighboring state, who tried the same thing in Bombay. It seems all her life she'd bathed with nothing but clay, so when she first went to Bombay, she continued as she always had done, though she lived on the fifth floor of an apartment building. Her maids were sent downstairs in the lift every day to fetch earth from the garden for her bath. This went on until the pipes became so clogged that the plumbing in the whole building broke down.

In those circumstances, she would have been better off to use chickpea flour, as we did sometimes, instead of mud. Chickpea flour, mixed with a bit of yogurt or water, makes a paste which really cleans the skin and leaves it silky soft, especially if you've had an oil massage first. Our maids would rub it repeatedly so it sort of crumbled off your skin, taking away all the deep-down dirt with it. This sounds painful but it wasn't. Sometimes we scrubbed extra hard with the dried fibers of a particular gourd, which Miss Blake said was like a loofah. That cleaned very well and it came from the palace gardens, so getting one was not a problem.

Our bathing routine in my father's palace was much the same as in Madanpur after my marriage, though by the time my second daughter was born, the bathrooms had all been renovated and we had running water throughout the palace. I must be a romantic because I regretted that a bit.

My favorite memories are of the big, steaming *hamams* and *ghangals* in the old-fashioned bathrooms.

Surely the most exotic bath I ever had in my life had nothing to do with modern plumbing; it was like something in the middle ages. I went with a friend in Bombay to the old Persian *hamam* or public bathing cavern that her family sometimes used. My friend was Muslim, so apart from the strangeness of bathing in the *hamam*, there was the fascination of learning her customs, which were different from those I knew as a Hindu. Her family had booked the *hamam* in advance and sent maids ahead of time to scrub it out thoroughly, as it was actually a public bathing place. They took their own towels and a big pot of henna or *mehndi* paste, which had been soaking all night. They also took huge hampers of food because we reached there about nine-thirty in the morning and didn't leave until late afternoon.

here were more than a dozen of us: my friend's mother, sisters, aunts, and cousins all came along, as well as their personal maids. The *hamam* was in an old section of the city, so to reach it we went down a narrow twisting alley and through a little door; it was like going into a cave. There was one big room, very dimly lit, and a smaller room off to one side. Two tanks of water sat there, one hot and one cold. The hot water tank had a sort of furnace underneath it. Wood could be fed into this furnace from outside the *hamam* and the fire could be stoked through the night. That way when we came to bathe in the morning, the water was quite hot and steamy.

The big bathing room was slightly raised in the center with drains running around its edges. There were little low platforms covered in tiles. These were for sitting and bathing; other longer ones were for stretching out while the maids massaged every square inch of our bodies. The whole room was tiled in those funny mosaic chips that you can look at without seeing for hours. The first thing we did was strip and put our clothes in the little room next to the tanks. One or two of us younger ones felt shy at first, but my friend's aunt teased us: "there are no menfolk here; why cover yourselves? Are we not made from the very same mold?"

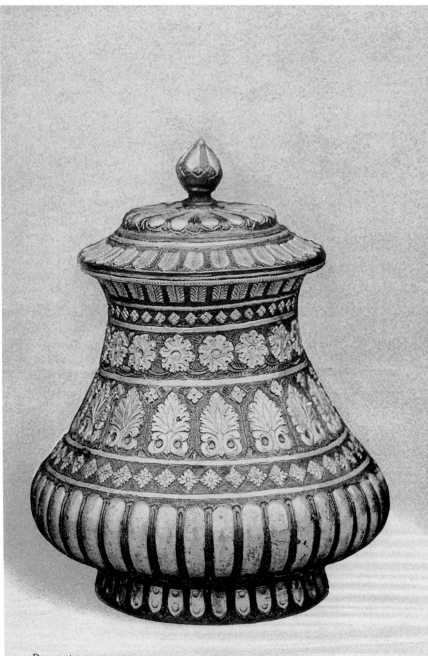

Decorative water pots

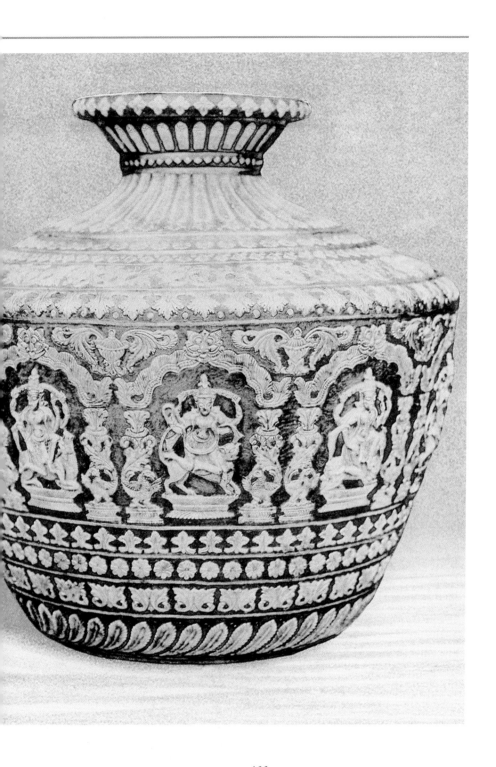

And so we relaxed and let the maids go to work. They rubbed the *mehndi* into our long hair, then wrapped our heads in a very thin cloth. Next we did something I had never done before; we poured a very watery paste of *mehndi* all over our bodies and left it on for fifteen minutes or so. When we rinsed this paste off, our skin had a wonderful olive glow that was different from the effect of the turmeric water I had sometimes used in Rajasthan. By the time all this was done, lunch was laid out and we tucked into the tiffin boxes right there in the middle of the room. After lunch we stretched out on the long stone slabs and chatted while the maids straightened things up and nibbled something themselves. I remember the gossip on that particular day: they were all excited about the wonderful miracle that had happened to my friend's sister. It couldn't be explained by modern science, they said.

The girl in question had a phantom pregnancy the first year of her marriage. The lady doctor had told her that she would never conceive: something was wrong with her womb. So she resorted to prayer and pilgrimages to holy places and holy men like so many Indian women. "We warned her about some of these sham holy men and their evil intentions," said my friends. Finally she met an old *pir*, a Muslim holy man who assured her that she would conceive if she followed his advice very strictly. He told her to eat one dried date fruit every single night for one hundred nights and only then lie with her husband. Well, she had followed his instructions faithfully. "You won't believe this," my friends said, "but she became pregnant right then. She's had a beautiful son and now she's taken him on a pilgrimage to our holy city of Karballa; just as the *pir* instructed." Miss Blake smiled at this when I told her but I believed them! Hadn't my wonderful banyan tree helped me to conceive?

Be that as it may, gossip gave way slowly to drowsiness and we were half asleep when the maids came back. They brought bowls of *sheera* with them. This *sheera* was really caramelized sugar, cooked to the consistency of very soft putty; it was used to remove unwanted body hair. I

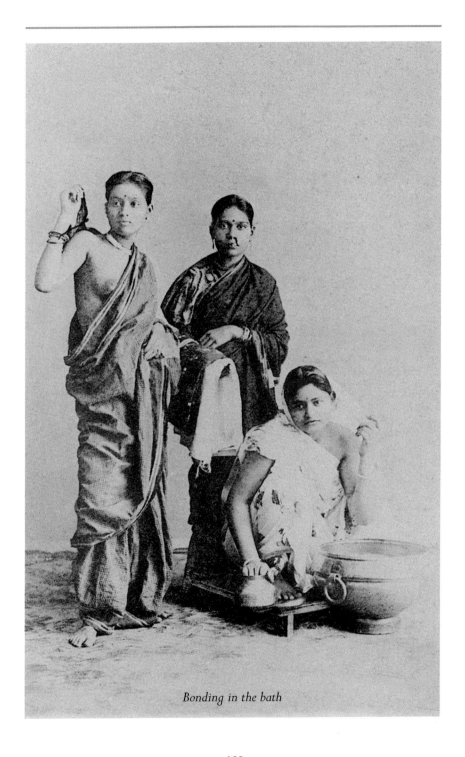

Bonding in the bath

had never seen this method used before. Because of the long treatments I had undergone as a child, I had no problems with superfluous hair. I had seen some of the ladies in Madanpur remove hair with hot ash, or ash mixed with chickpea flour or sugar syrup. But this *sheera* was made from a cup of sugar and the juice of two limes cooked on a low flame until the sugar caramelized; then it was cooled and rolled into a ball. The maids placed the putty on a hairy area, spread it out with their fingers and then pulled it off together with the unwanted hairs. They repeated the process until all the hair was removed.

The maids began to scrub us then, using a loofah-like *kheesa*. They scrubbed long and slowly: the dirt literally rolled off. Then we washed. Just as in our *zenana*, my Muslim friends didn't use soap; they used something called *safidaab* from Iran. Someone said it was pellets of sun-dried sheep's fat. I don't know. It looked very dry and white and it had to be rubbed around and around on a stone like we rub sandalwood sticks to make paste. The maids rubbed this *safidaab* paste on our necks, arms, and faces. Still more dirt came away, but after that *safidaab* treatment we were all soft and shiny and I noticed it wasn't the least bit drying like our chickpea flour can be.

My friend told me much later that when they stopped getting regular supplies of *safidaab* from Iran, their father made them use pure almond oil on their skin and also drink a teaspoon of it at night. He said it kept their faces smooth and soft. Once in a while they put a few strands of saffron in the oil to give a little flattering glow to the skin.

But back to the *hamam*. When the scrubbing was finished, it was time to rinse the henna out of our hair. This took buckets of water and lots of combing, but the sweet smell of *mehndi* lingered for days. We didn't use any soap at all, even on our bodies—just *safidaab*, scrubbing, and water.

I noticed some of the women do a little ritual called *ghusul*, signifying the end of the bath. While they said a short prayer, they poured just a little bit of water, first over the head, then over the right shoulder and finally over the left shoulder. My friend told me they do this in the belief that an angel sits on either shoulder. They take that angel's name while pouring the water. I couldn't understand why the other women were teasing those doing the *ghusul*. Then my friend explained that when a woman performs the *ghusul* it usually means she has lain with her husband the previous night. Muslim law requires her to perform the *ghusul* after sex or when she has finished her periods.

When all the sluicing and scrubbing and slippery work was over, it was almost four o'clock: time for tea. So we wrapped ourselves in thin, absorbent towels, very much like the *panchas* or *gamchas*, which I use to this day, and we settled down to the business of tea before returning to the everyday world. When the tea was over, those of us who had the courage took a final dip in very cold water before dressing and slipping away.

That was the end of my most exotic bath, but I saw another fascinating *hamam* once, in a Kashmiri friend's home. It was a large room with four long, flat stones. These stones were heated by a wood fire, which burned in an underground cellar beneath the room. By lying down on those stones, a person could foment her back and waist. This was supposed to be very beneficial for women after childbirth. Following this fomentation, you went into an adjoining room and bathed yourself with water which had been heated by the same wood fire. That was a Kashmiri *hamam*.

The most unusual and practical bathroom I've seen was in South India. Almost every home there had a *handa* in the bathroom, a large copper vessel cemented in the ground. This had a wooden lid that was lifted to fill it with water and to remove it when it was heated. Below the *handa* was a wood fire that could be fed with all the rubbish from the garden and the kitchen, so it was a practical as well as a pleasant *hamam*.

There is a sweet little custom I have always followed after bathing and dressing in the morning. I do it to this day as do many Indian women; it gives me a wonderful feeling of contentment. The custom is called *tulsi puja*. In the courtyard of a traditional Hindu home, there was always a little raised square planter, like a chimney said Miss Blake, nicely whitewashed. In this grew the sacred *tulsi* or basil plant which we worship every morning as Lakshmi, pouring a bit of water on the plant from a brass *lota* as we circle it slowly, saying a

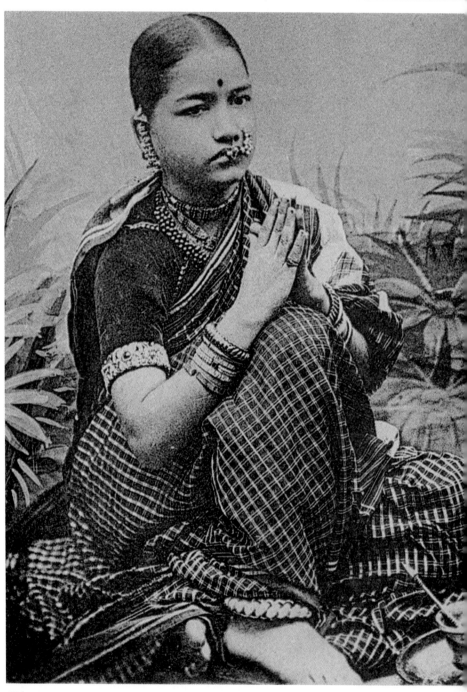

Tulsi puja

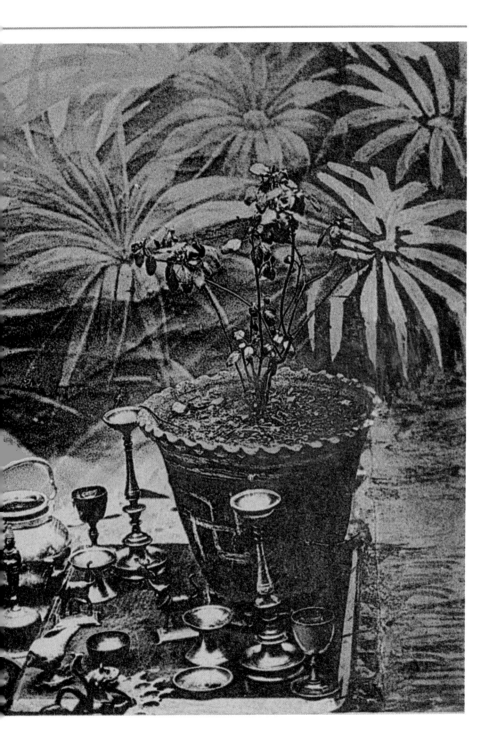

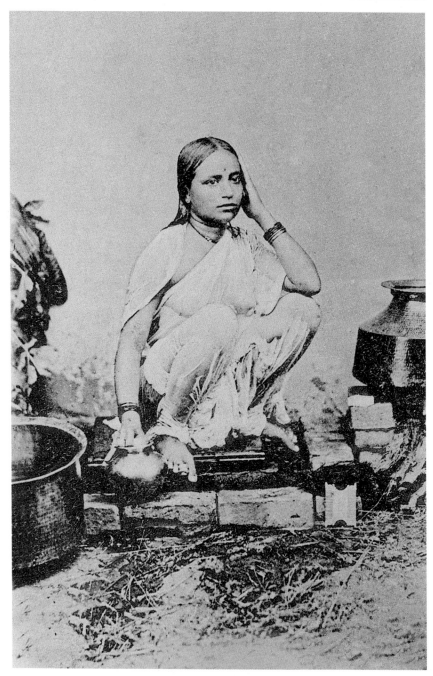

Heating the bath water

prayer. I do that to this day, though my plant is in a pot now, I don't feel my day will go well without having paid my respects to the *tulsi*. We believe this little *puja* protects our home and family and makes Lakshmi look with favor on us. In fact, we seem to have a reverence for many natural things, which borders on a sort of worship.

I have always loved the benediction which says, "May you remain as pure as the basil, may the members of your family constantly bloom like the banana, may they prosper like the *durva* grass, may they achieve the serenity of the banyan and the *peepal*, and may all their sorrows be carried away by the river Ganges."

They are like our friends, these useful gifts of nature, helping us in our pursuit of beauty, health, and happiness. One of our proverbs says, "nothing on earth can compare with the virtues of the basil." Our people say that if you plant a *tulsi* near your home, the atmosphere is purified. I know that as a home remedy, basil leaf juice is used for curing fevers, hiccups, coughs, and colds and even for loss of appetite. It's always been a favorite remedy of mine for curing the children's sore throats. I would brew it with lemon grass, coriander seeds, and anise in three cups of water mixed with rock candy and let it cook until reduced to one-third. The decoction always fixed their throats.

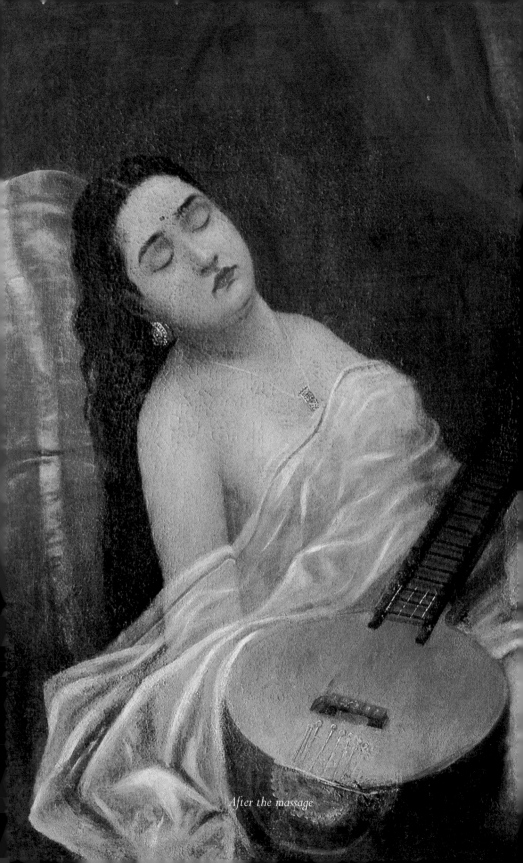

After the massage

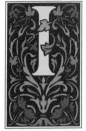

7

Indulging the Body

As a young girl, I had a similar feeling of contentment lying in bed at night, almost asleep, while a drowsy maid rubbed the soles of my feet with a *kasha katori*. *Kasha* is an alloy of five auspicious metals. A *katori* is a little bowl, smooth and round at the bottom, just big enough to fit in your hand. The maid would dip this little bowl in clarified butter and rub the smooth bottom of that buttery bowl against the soles of my feet until I slept. This was my parents' idea; they said it kept the feet soft and supple, but more importantly, it drew the heat out of young, growing bodies, so that one's nature remained calm and composed.

I thought my parents were just indulging me with this rubbing; but years later in Madanpur, Pandit Dubey once recommended this very process for removing the heat from my body when I had a high fever. It had to be done with a special clarified butter called *shataghrita*, which means "beaten with one hundred strokes." He said the process would be soothing for my eyes as well and of course he quoted this verse from *Charak* to me: "By massaging the feet, roughness, immobility, dryness, fatigue and numbness are instantaneously cured; tenderness, strength and steadiness of feet are effected, the eyesight becomes clear and *vata*, the vital cell-force in the body is thereby relieved." My fever disappeared very quickly and I was not really surprised.

You see, whether it be feet or faces, fingers or heads, Indians believe very strongly in the benefits of massage. I think that's true in the whole of the country, though of course the techniques differ and ingredients for massage vary from region to region. I have already spoken of how I was massaged as a bride to make my skin soft and sweet-smelling and as a new mother to strengthen my muscles and increase the circulation. I have also mentioned how babies are massaged to keep their little limbs limber and supple and their spines in perfect alignment. The massage process continues throughout one's life—if you are lucky, that is.

We believe in massage for so many reasons: to maintain muscle tone and increase blood circulation, to stay supple and slim, to keep the skin soft and sweet-smelling, and to keep it free of hair, not to speak of the sheer pleasure of the process. Maybe we're a nation of hedonists! I remember once reading some Englishman's memoirs recorded in the eighteenth century. He wrote about the inhabitants of a small Indian town he visited and said that in the afternoon "they stretch themselves upon a sopha, where they were kneaded like dough." He went on to say that "the necessity of promoting the circulation of the fluids, too often retarded by the heat of the climate, first suggested the notion of this operation, which affords them infinite variety of sensations. They fall into such a tender state of languor that they sometimes almost faint away!"

I must say, I have never fainted away, but to this day I enjoy my massage. It helps to have maids pummel and pound you; but massage is quite possible without anything more than a loving friend to help. In a pinch, one can even massage oneself adequately enough to keep the skin soft and supple. You need only understand which oils to use in which seasons, what the properties of these oils are, and when to apply them. Creams can never compare with oils no matter how rich they may be. They just do not have the same effect on the body.

Of course, my granddaughter teases me. She claims that if women in the West used my beauty treatment, they would need to have kitchen utensils on their dressing tables instead of pretty bottles and jars!

I suppose she's right. You would need graters and mixers, a grinding stone and a burner, and perhaps a little mortar and pestle too, if you were to prepare everything fresh as we did in the days when I was a girl. But today many of the oils are available in bottles, as are the turmeric and chickpea powders and even some of the *utanas* or *uptanas*. *Utanas* are the ground spices and condiments that we use both to perfume and to cleanse our bodies. They are such a lovely invention, everyone should know about them.

Some are available ready-made in India; but others must be handmade. Take for example this recipe, which I recently sent to Miss Blake's daughter for a skin treatment. Soak a half cup of almonds overnight and remove their skins the next morning. Grind them to a fine paste with half a cup of whole milk, then simmer over very low heat until the almonds emit that special rich aroma which tells you they're releasing their oils. Let this paste cool. Add a pinch of saffron threads, which have been carefully powdered in a mortar and pestle. Mix well and rub the paste over your face and body. Let it dry while you relax. Then sit in the shower or tub and slowly rub the dry paste off your body. It will leave you all clean, soft, and sweet-smelling.

This was one of our favorite *utanas* in Madanpur. The maids used to remove it by first dipping their hands in a little jasmine oil, then rubbing us from head to toe. But I personally had a preference for a different *utana* made of coconut, which we always used in my mother's house when I was young. It was made by boiling freshly grated coconut with a pinch of saffron and a little turmeric powder. The oil that resulted was particularly good during winter months when our skin became dry from the cold. Mind you, it was a relative cold, nothing like the cold in Kashmir. There they use an *utana* of chickpea flour and yogurt mixed in equal proportions with orange peel that has been dried and powdered. These ingredients are mixed with enough oil to make a paste, and then rubbed into the skin and left for fifteen minutes before they are rinsed with warm water.

Our real problem in Rajasthan was not the cold, but the heat. So we used a lot of sandalwood on our faces and bodies. Apart from its fragrance, sandalwood is known to have cooling properties and also to prevent prickly heat. Sandalwood reminds me of another *utana* I occasionally used, one I learned in South India. Lightly grease a heavy iron griddle and heat the following ingredients: a half cup each of black onion seed, white mustard seed,

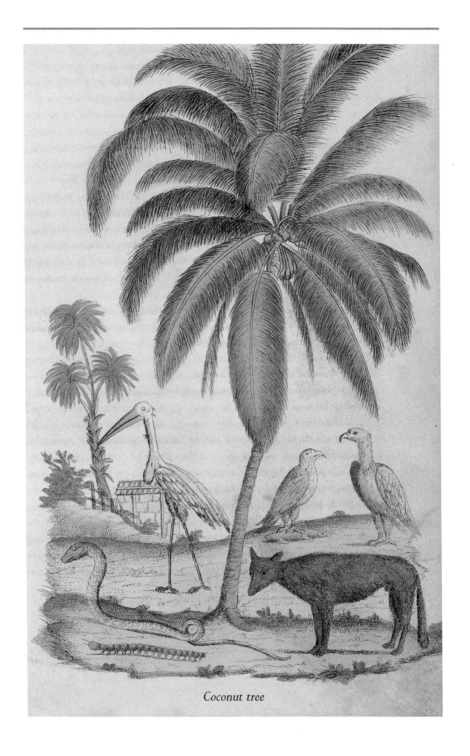

Coconut tree

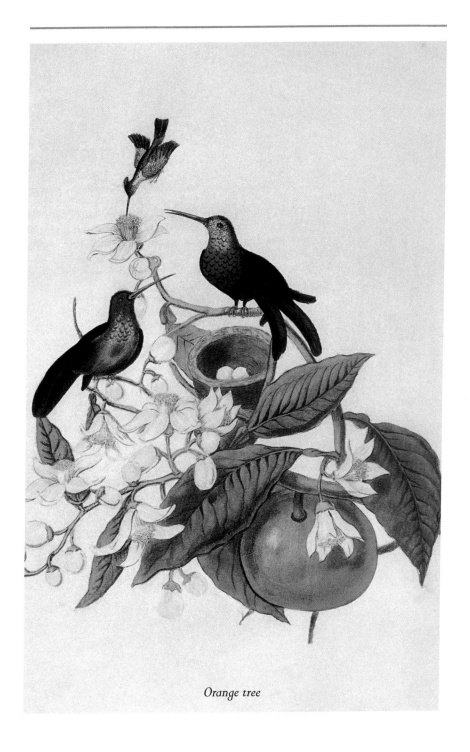

Orange tree

grated coconut, and dried orange peel. When all these ingredients begin to release their aroma, remove them from the griddle and grind them fine in a blender. Then add enough water to make a fairly thick paste and grind again until thoroughly blended. You can store this *utana* in a tightly lidded jar. Use a quarter cup before bathing, rubbing it well into the skin and rinsing it off thoroughly.

There are so many *utanas*. This one from Maharashtra is more like a deep cleanser, though it is said to be cooling as well. Soak equal parts of barley and gram in water until they can be easily ground to a paste. Bake this paste in a slow oven until it is golden and crumbles easily. Then rub this coarse flour into the skin. It acts almost like a soft pumice stone to remove skin that is dead or roughened.

he most auspicious time of the year for *utanas* is Diwali, a festival usually in October or November. It signifies the end of the monsoon and the beginning of winter. We welcome Lakshmi, the goddess of wealth, into our home at Diwali. It is a time when people not only do their accounts but also undertake their major housecleaning and household repairs. At Diwali, men too must, by tradition, take a ritual *utana* rubbing and bath.

In Madanpur a huge silver tray would be brought both to the *zenana* and to the men's quarters on the morning of Diwali. It held dozens of small silver bowls. These bowls contained every possible ingredient for a fragant *utana*: paste of almond and sandalwood, pastes made from lentils, turmeric, and saffron powders or even chickpea flour. There were also jasmine and other fragrant oils, ground poppy seeds and sesame seeds, and *shikakai* and *ritha* for hair washing. The children had a ball with all these goodies, smearing themselves, laughing, splashing, scrubbing, and teasing each other mercilessly, and even getting clean in the bargain.

Women were slightly more sober about it. Many of us took the Diwali massage and bath quite seriously, treating it as a sort of ritual. These rituals went on for five days before the actual day of the festival. They were per-

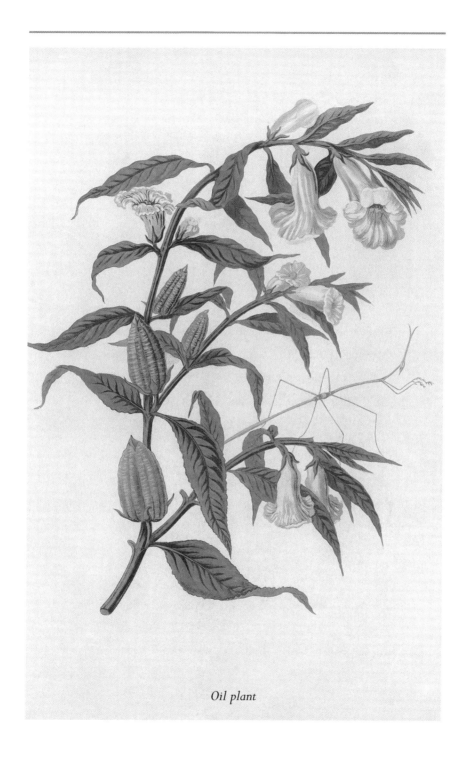

Oil plant

formed like a prayer to ensure the prosperity of our home during that year. When I was still in my mother's house, we used to make beautiful designs at Diwali to decorate our *bajots* or *chaurangs*, the big low stools on which we would sit while our women massaged and rubbed us with *utanas*. My mother traced elaborate patterns of *rangoli* or *alpana* around the *bajot* with white and colored rice powder.

My massage woman had her own way of rendering that spot auspicious. She would dip the fingertips of her right hand into the bowl of coconut oil with which she was soon to massage me. Ever so carefully, she marked the earth around the stool with five spots of oil. Then with her index finger she put a sixth spot in the center to ward off that dreaded evil eye. Only then did she put the oil first on my hair, working it slowly down along my hands and legs, back and chest, always massaging firmly toward the heart, just as the woman who later massaged me after childbirth was careful to do. At the end of it all, she would put a little extra oil in my navel and say, "There," with great satisfaction. "That's where your life began, little one, right at the spot—so don't rub that oil, leave it there."

In my mother's house, we used coconut oil for the massage. Though coconuts were uncommon in Rajasthan, my mother had a preference for them. So each week a bullock-cart full of coconuts arrived at the palace from somewhere on the coast west of our state. On Sundays, the household maids sat in groups, breaking open these coconuts and grating them to make the oil. The graters were lovely; we called them *kisnis*. They were made of brass in many different shapes like parrots, peacocks, and turtles. Each was cleverly designed so the animal's little serrated beak or tail could scrape out the coconut from the inside. When their work was over, the maids squeezed all the milk from the grated coconut into big cooking vessels. That coconut milk was boiled until the oil floated to the surface. Then that oil was skimmed and kept for massage.

Sometimes they added turmeric powder if the oil was for the body and not for a head massage. The turmeric rhizomes were first pounded in a big mortar and then ground to a powder on the stone hand mill, just like the one

I used during my pregnancies to strengthen my spine. The women who turned the mill used to sing. I can hear them to this day: "Let's turn the hand mill. It's not a strenuous task. Since mother wisely brought me up on tonics of nutmeg and sweetflag. Which makes my arms strong."

They would sit in a group under a big *peepal* tree on the women's side of the palace, or on the veranda during the monsoons, laughing and chatting as they split those coconuts and grated them vigorously. How I loved that laughter, that feeling of belonging. Even if I watched it from afar, I knew we were sisters and mothers and daughters to each other; there was never a doubt about that.

You know, those days are gone; but even here in Bombay, though I live alone, I know I have only to go out of my door to find sisters galore if I seek them. We're a funny lot we Indian women; we chat with one another quite naturally: no need for an introduction. My granddaughter finds this very strange. It's not that way in her America. But here, women share at the drop of a hat: on a train, on a bus, walking down the road, we just talk as though it were the most natural thing. Today it is not hard for me to recapture that friendly feeling of my father's palace even here in this big, busy city.

When I married, I changed not only locations but traditions as well. My husband's family was a strong believer in the benefits of mustard oil. "It penetrates the body and warms the muscles like no other oil," they assured me. "Just look at the small princes' gymnastics teacher." A splendid young wrestler from Punjab, he trained the boys to massage themselves in mustard oil before their exercises. He also made them dance on his back to work the oil into his muscles. "Has it not done them a world of good?" my new relatives pointed out proudly.

"And what about mustard oil's antiseptic properties? Everyone knows that all pickled foods are best kept in mustard oil." That was another argument in favor of the oil. There was a story of the nearby school involving mustard oil and the measles epidemic. According to my family, when the measles broke out, there was a fear that the infection might spread to the

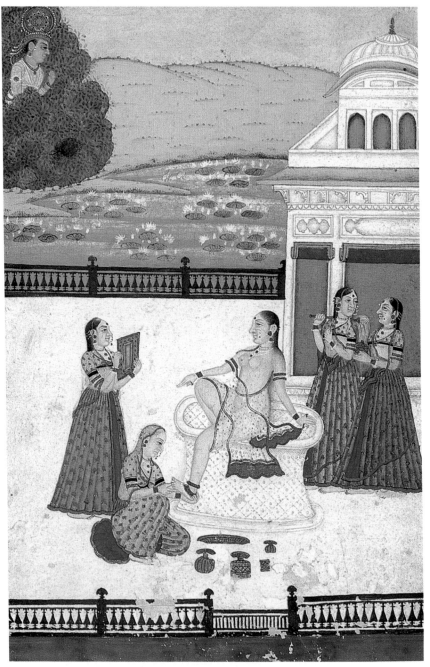

Indulging in massage

state troops who were encamped nearby. So their commandant ordered every soldier to keep his nostrils lightly coated with mustard oil. And believe it or not, his tactics succeeded. Not one case of measles was reported in the cantonment. Another case touting the virtues of mustard oil! Even Chhoti-Ma was forever recommending a paste of mustard oil mixed with turmeric powder for any fungus infection on the body, particularly if you got it between your toes.

I could not refute all their good arguments, but I just did not like mustard oil. Its smell and taste were too foreign to me. I was used to coconut oil for massage and sesame oil for cooking. Much to my husband's disappointment, I couldn't even eat all the palace dishes that were prepared in their favorite oil. So, though my mother had advised me to obey always, I had to insist on my coconut oil for massage and on sesame oil or clarified butter for cooking. Badi-Ma took this as a sign of rebellion, but no one else seemed to mind much. Habits do vary after all.

I noticed, for example, that in South India, people swear by the virtues of *til* or sesame oil. There, women normally have their oil massage and bath on a Tuesday or Friday. Those are also the days on which the goddesses Amba and Parvati are worshipped. So you see, customs differ everywhere.

 think it was Pandit Dubey who told me that "shampoo" was originally an Indian word. It didn't mean washing your hair, but came from the verb *champna*, "to knead and press the muscles of the body to relieve fatigue." Of course *Charak* had something to say on the matter and the Pandit quoted it with great relish: "The body of one who practices oil massage regularly is not much injured, even if subjected to injuries and strenuous work; his physique is smooth, strong and charming. With regular oil massage the onslaught of ageing is slackened." My maids get the giggles when I quote that one to them while they are rubbing oil on me!

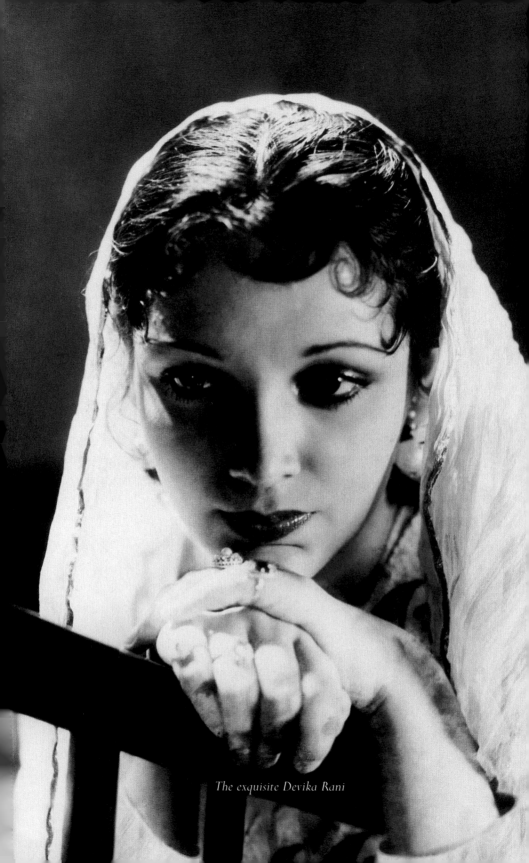

The exquisite Devika Rani

8.

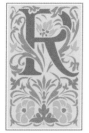

Radiant Complexion

I am sorry to tell you that these maids of mine tease me. They say, "Mother, why do you carry on with this massage and for whom do you make yourself lovely? Is there a man in your life? You know mother, marrying an old woman is like begging from a beggar: there isn't much you can get out of it." Imagine! They say such things to me! As though they themselves are dewy-eyed babes, when they've been with me since the day of my marriage.

Actually we all carry on with these rituals, both my naughty maids and I, because the rituals themselves are old friends by now. The massage, the bath, the various shampoos and conditioners, the *utanas*; they are so much a part of life, we would be lonely if we left all that behind. I know they say that a man at sixty is a bull elephant, and a woman of twenty is already on the decline; but that doesn't mean we give up in despair and abandon our beauty routines. In the first place, our makeup was never much more than careful grooming, bright eyes, and a smile. We didn't use cosmetics or anything too obvious or brazen. In those days they didn't exist; and later when they did, our husbands and families made it clear we were not to use them. "Humility pleases everyone" was the motto and that meant in makeup as well.

It was the same for all of us, so we didn't mind. And frankly to this day, though I'm perfectly free to do as I like, I cannot fool around with those bottles and jars. There is something to be said for continuity, for treating one's assets consistently and not subjecting them to the whims of fashion. Most women of my age have followed the same simple beauty routines and used the same natural products from their earliest childhood. Their makeup and the way they care for their faces are no exception.

I say "makeup," but I should really say, their "facial adornment" because for an Indian woman of my generation, each embellishment has a meaning or a purpose beyond beautification and certainly apart from anything to do with fashion. At least that was the case in my younger days. My granddaughter's look is different, much more modern. But we were very simple. We wore red powder in the parting of our hair, a dot of color in the center of our foreheads, *kaajal* or lampblack in our eyes, and a bit of red on our lips, but that redness came from *paan*, not from lipstick. Sometimes we put a bit of color in our cheeks by mixing the same red powder we used on our foreheads with a little clarified butter, then rubbing this on our cheekbones. That was the extent of our makeup.

"A fair face needs no paint" was the general belief and, "Who has a good nature has a good face," was the maxim my mother used to quote to reassure me as we looked into the mirror together. Now that did not mean we didn't care for ourselves. Goodness, no! We spent hours preparing face packs for our skin, special *kaajals* for our eyes, and various *paans* to stain our mouths the plesasing red color that Miss Blake found so unattractive.

Let me start with skin care. First of all I must say that when I was a girl, hardly anyone I knew had pimples. I don't know why that was; perhaps as the magazines all say today, it had something to do with eating natural foods and using only natural products. I'm sure it also had to do with our lifestyle in those days, which was relatively free from tension. If occasionally a pimple did crop up, Pandit Dubey or one of his associates would brew us an herbal tea to cleanse our systems. Then, of course, various ladies from the *zenana* would come forward with their pet remedies for flawless skin.

My favorite remedy for pimples was *am haldi* or *ambia haldi, Curcuma amada* to Pandit Dubey. *Am haldi* has many of the same purifying and astringent qualities as ginger but ginger is "heating," whereas *am haldi* is "cooling," which is what you want when you have skin eruptions. I taught my own daughters this *am haldi* treatment which they have used all of their lives. Take a teaspoon of *am haldi* turmeric powder and one or two strands of saffron, powder them in a little mortar and pestle, then add a teaspoon of fresh, unboiled milk and mix this powder into a paste. Apply this paste on the eruptions and leave for about an hour. Doing this every day will heal them so thoroughly that no mark will be left on the face.

Am haldi is a distant cousin of *jungli haldi* or Cochin *haldi*, which is a kind of wild turmeric used by the famous Kathakali dancers of Kerala. These dancers have to use a great deal of makeup while performing their pageants. Wild turmeric is the only thing they have found which can protect their faces from the harmful effects of this makeup over a long period of time. But plain turmeric from the grocer's can be substituted for its more exotic cousins. All the members of the turmeric family are good for removing skin discolorations, or reducing swelling from bruises or sprains. I have already mentioned its other medicinal properties: how good turmeric is as an antiseptic, how quickly it healed my poor maid's chin when it had a severe cut.

Many people believe in turmeric for the skin; others swear by a commonly available earth called *multani mitti*. Miss Blake identified *multani mitti* as Fuller's earth. We use this crumbly, gray-yellow clay in place of soap. It is also very effective for pimples. Take a pinch of it in your palm, add a few drops of water and dab this paste onto the pimple. When it dries, peel it off and put on another layer. It will dry up the pimple, but never discolor the skin like some modern products I know. Many women in India have never used any cleansing agent on their faces but *multani mitti*.

One of Bombay's greatest beauties, who is now as young as I, has always used a face pack made of rose water mixed with *multani mitti*. Before a party she lies down with this mask on her face and cucumber slices pressed on her eyelids. The effect is remarkable; her face looks so smooth and fresh. I tried it once or twice but could never keep from chatting and thus cracking the mask; she is a quieter type.

A substitute for *multani mitti* is chickpea flour or *besan*, the same flour some women use on their bodies for a bath. You must be careful, however,

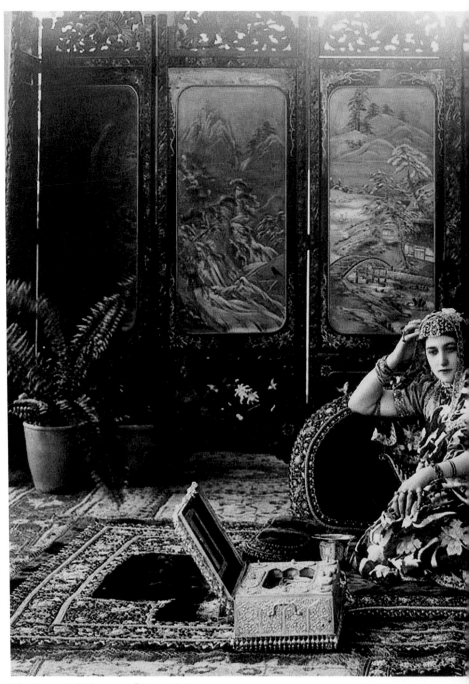

The Spanish Maharani of Kapurthala

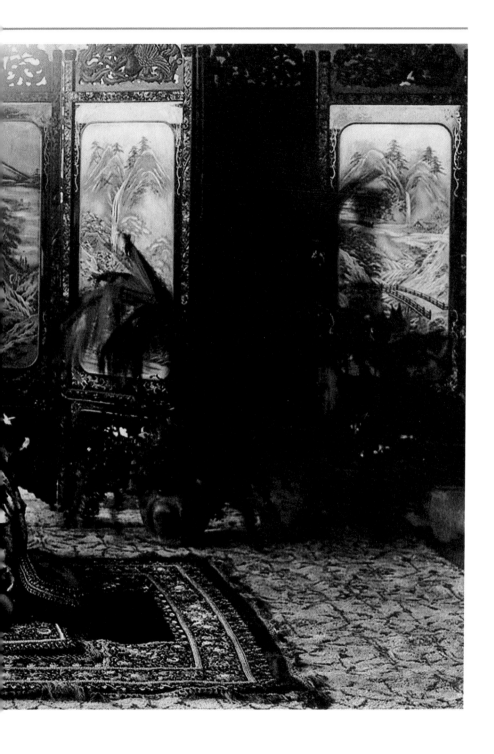

because this flour is drying, so for dry skins it is better to use it mixed with a little milk or cream. Many of the *utanas* women use in the bath can also be used on the face. Almonds are particularly useful. Instead of buying expensive almond creams, I just take one or two blanched almonds, rub them on a clear, rough surface moistened with a little water. This makes a paste which can be rubbed on the face and left to dry thoroughly. When it is dry, rub it off gently with the tips of the fingers, which have been dipped in water. All the dirt and dry skin will come away.

Another nut, the pistachio, is good for dark circles under the eyes. This is a problem Indian women seem to have more often than fair skinned ladies. We grind a few pistachio nuts with a teaspoon of milk and gently apply this to the delicate area around the eyes. Then we wash it off after half an hour. Like so many natural remedies, this one doesn't work overnight: it takes time and patience. That is why consistency is so important. Women of my generation understood this and were careful to impart to their daughters not only the remedy but also an understanding of why and how it works, so they will not be tempted to abandon it in haste.

I remember that in our dowry trousseaus we were given little red sandalwood dolls, which were actually to be used on our skin. Their bodies were made of a variety of sandalwood called *rakta-chandan*, which you rubbed on a rough stone with a little water. The reddish paste that resulted was good for so many things: pimples, skin allergies, rashes, and swellings. Just imagine— there was that little doll, tucked into our enormous dowry chests, along with our wedding *saris*, linen, and jewelry, as a loving reminder from the women of our families to look after our skin.

As I said, every woman in the *zenana* had a different remedy. These *zenana* women came in marriage from many regions of India so their ideas of beauty care and the ingredients they used were very diverse. My own mother-in-law, of course, was devoted to mustard. She even used it on her face, soaking a few mustard seeds in water overnight and then grinding them in the morning with a teaspoon of milk and a quarter teaspoon of turmeric powder. She claimed this paste would deal with any pimple.

A distant aunt, who had a lovely complexion, used to make a paste of one or two almonds, a teaspoon of poppy seeds, a teaspoon of milk, and a quarter teaspoon of turmeric powder. She would put this on her face every day before her bath, and she never had so much as one blemish. But for those who did, she had a pet remedy: grind together whole black lentils, which we call *masoor*, with a little clarified butter and milk. "Apply this to the face for seven days and see the results," she would say.

ne of my grandmothers-in-law, who also had flawless skin, never applied anything at all on her face. Her secret was that she ate a pinch of powdered *vekhand* every single night—just a quarter gram of the bitter herb sweetened with honey. She claimed it aided her digestion. Miss Blake identified *vekhand* as sweetflag. Sweetflag was always stocked in the *zenana* under Pandit Dubey's instructions because it was effective in a number of children's ailments like indigestion, loss of appetite, coughs, and colds. A couple of rounds on the special rubbing stone with a little milk would do the trick.

I have found that throughout India there is a very strong faith in dairy products, an ingrained belief that any product that comes from the sacred cow is naturally soothing and beneficial to human beings. Look how yogurt is used as a hair conditioner and clarified butter for softening the feet. Or think about the village woman. She has no such thing as a night cream. She simply boils the fresh milk from the cow every evening and uses the *khurchan*, the cream from the bottom of the pot, to rub into her face before sleeping.

One of the most common face masks used by Indian women consists of three dairy products: yogurt, milk, and *ghee* or clarified butter, mixed with a bit of honey. Half a teaspoon of each makes an excellent mask to be left on the face for about twenty minutes. It's amazing how the richness of dairy products can prevent premature wrinkling.

Honey by itself is also very good for the complexion. Add half an egg to a tablespoon of honey and beat the two until they are creamy. This makes a good mask for normal skin. I get a bit hungry just thinking about it: honey is

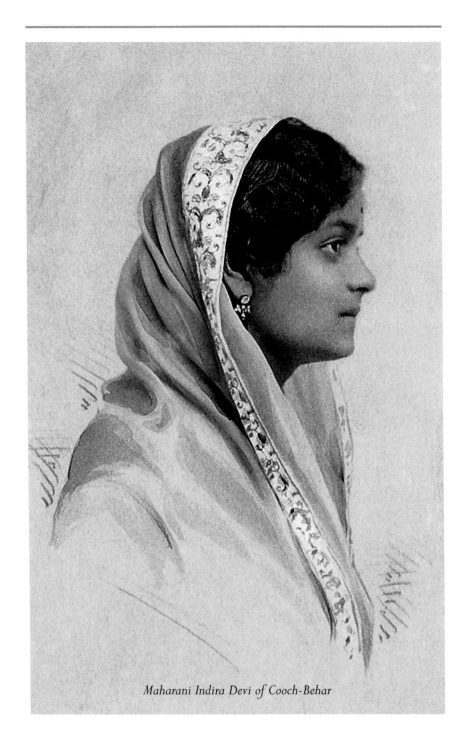

Maharani Indira Devi of Cooch-Behar

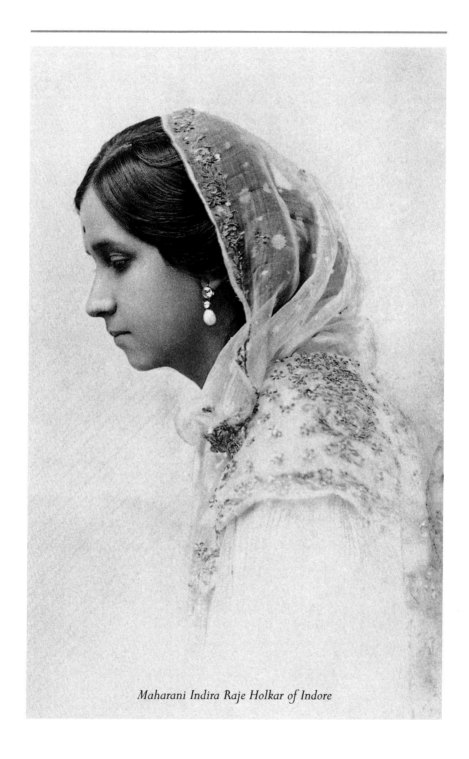

Maharani Indira Raje Holkar of Indore

a favorite of mine. Like my mother, I have always kept a good supply of it in the house: honey has so many uses. We used to give it to the children when their appetites waned, mixed with some clarified butter. A bit of this mixture, morning and evening, always seemed to revive those appetites quickly. Perhaps that is why we give tiny newborn babies a bit of honey on their tongues during the *jatkarma sanskar* ceremony, when the child's father dips a gold coin in honey and clarified butter and puts it on his little one's tongue.

I have already mentioned the veneration we have for natural things. Look at all the trees and plants we Hindus revere. They're all medicinal and useful: the basic *durva* grass, the *peepal*, banyan and *neem* trees, the *shami*, banana, *bael,* and *mandar.* All of them help to keep us healthy and therefore beautiful.

Among natural things, the rose is perhaps a bit more exotic than butter or banana trees! But the rose, too, has its place in beauty care. We were lucky in Madanpur to have a rose garden. The maids used to go out in the evening and gather fallen petals by the kilo, piling them into their big woven baskets, and carrying them off to soak overnight in huge earthen jars. These jars were kept near the bathing area of the *zenana* courtyard. In the morning many of us would go to those jars after bathing, squeeze out some petals and splash that fresh water on our faces. Some women swore that rose water was good not only for the complexion but also for the eyes, keeping them sparkling clear.

Petals of the fragrant, wild, pink rose were kept apart from the others especially to make *gulkand. Gulkand* was not exactly a beauty remedy; it was more of a cure-all, like the *leghyam* my South Indian friend used to keep next to her bed at all times. *Gulkand* was particularly good for constipation, so in that sense it kept the skin clear. We used to make big batches and keep them for the children. They always had a spoonful a day. *Gulkand* was made by layering rose petals with crystal sugar in a big, tightly lidded glass jar. This jar was then kept for fifteen days in the sun or in a very warm place. It had to mature another six weeks before we could begin to eat it, but never did children take

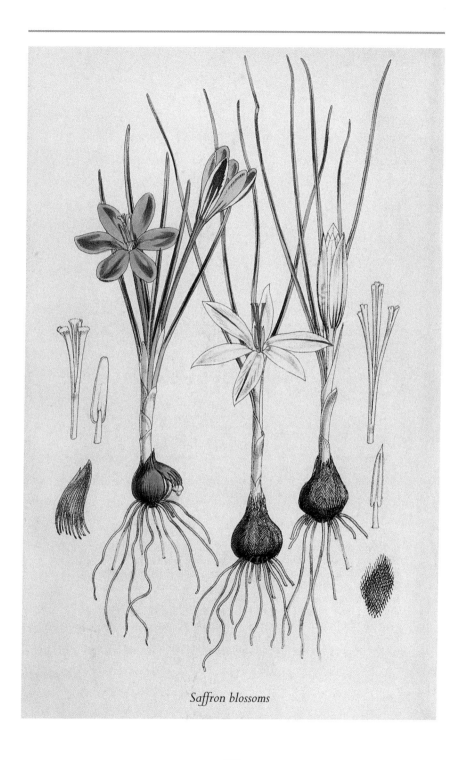

Saffron blossoms

a digestive so willingly as they did this beautiful and delicious *gulkand*, made of pure roses and sugar.

For the opposite problem of constipation, we used to give the children nutmeg. That was Chhoti-Ma's remedy, I remember. She used to warn against giving too much: an overdose could make you feel inebriated. "Just a quarter gram," she said. "Rub it on a marble surface and mix with a little clarified butter, that should do the trick very quickly." You can add sugar or honey to disguise the taste, if the children find nutmeg too strong.

Chhoti-Ma was thoughtful of everyone, but especially children. I am sorry to say that another relative who lived in the palace was much less sensitive to children's feelings. I shall not name her; suffice it to say that we always called her "The Lovely One," and not fondly. She was the one woman I could not abide. You see, The Lovely One had a beautiful face, an exquisite complexion, but no kindness in her heart or face. Her dominant trait was vanity.

Sadly, the one who suffered was The Lovely One's own daughter, Rajani. Little Rajani, through no fault of her own, daily offended her mother's vanity, because Rajani's skin was not fair. Like her name, which means "the night," Rajani was dark; or at least darker than pleased her mother. The Lovely One used to scrub her and scrub her, trying to lighten her skin. Indians love nature, it is true, but some of us cannot accept Mother Nature's choice of skin color unless it is the palest of pales. Miss Blake used to think this was such a pity, especially when she herself was always out there in the women's courtyard, trying to make her pale skin darker.

My complexion is wheaten, so perhaps I'm prejudiced in my own favor, but I have always found darker skins so attractive. Jewelry looks wonderful against a dark background; the teeth seem to shine in one's face, and clothes take on a special allure. Miss Blake could never carry off color the way *zenana* women could. Rajani's mother could never see this. Her daughter had a wonderful carriage, beautiful eyes, and a smile that was full of sunshine, but that was not enough for The Lovely One, she wanted a milky skinned daughter. Sadly, many Indian women have this feeling. Even today, some women put rice flour or powder on their dark faces, trying to make them look paler.

y own parents never ever made me conscious of my wheaten complexion. But they did stress the need for a healthy diet, plenty of fruit, plenty of water, and regular exercise. My father taught me the *Surya Namaskar* exercise when I was six years old. That means I've been doing it for almost seventy years! *Surya Namaskar* is a yogic exercise. Literally it means "homage to the sun." It is really a series of movements strung together into one. Those movements exercise every important muscle and limb of one's body. Pandit Dubey seemed very pleased when I told him that I did this exercise regularly. He professed that *Surya Namaskar* effectively tones up the various glands in the body as well as the digestive, respiratory, and nervous systems. It may not keep you slim, but it will keep you supple. We in India find too much slimness disturbing, as though Lakshmi, the goddess of prosperity, had passed by that slim one's door at Diwali without going in. For us, pleasantly plump means pleasantly prosperous—at least for those of my generation.

As I have been saying all along, a woman, in the orthodox Indian way of thinking, is more than just herself; she is a representative of her husband and his family; she is literally the goddess Lakshmi in a way. Her demeanor, dress, and bodily adornment must reflect this status. There is a village proverb that goes, "If I am not to put this red spot on my forehead, how am I to please my husband?" Just as our plumpness tells the world that our family prospers, so our facial adornment does more than accent our beauty; it also signifies our marital status and many believe it has deeper meanings as well. Miss Blake did some research on this.

She found that the origins of the *tilak* or red spot that Hindu women wear on their foreheads has really been lost over the centuries, though scholars have several theories. Some say it dates back to pre-Aryan times, before peoples from the North swept through India and imposed their own customs

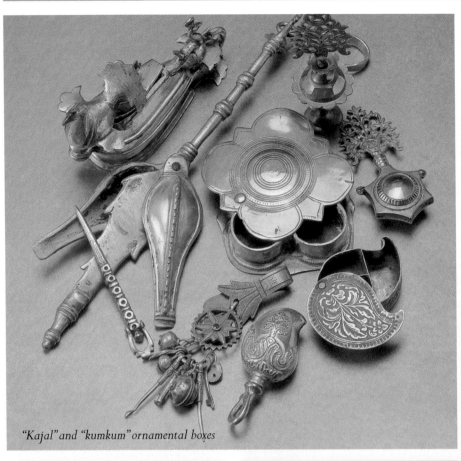

"Kajal" and "kumkum" ornamental boxes

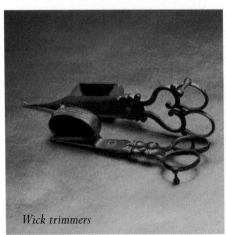

Wick trimmers

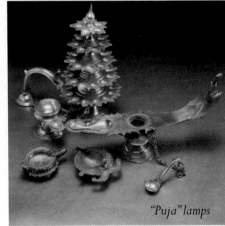

"Puja" lamps

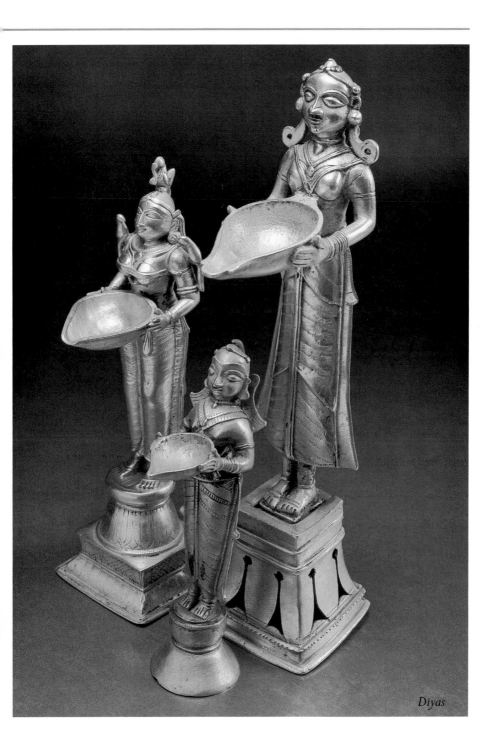

Diyas

and castes. They claim that when a man took his bride home, the custom was that he go hunting, kill an animal, and mark his new wife's forehead with a spot of its blood. Other scholars say that our *tilak* represents the third eye of Lord Shiva, the potent energy that has the power to destroy all evil forces. Whatever its origin, the *tilak* has become a custom with us. Any woman who is not a widow can put a spot on her forehead, though there are now many different "fashions" in spots, including little plastic ones that stick and restick and glittery ones that glow in the dark.

n my mother's days, a *tilak* was made of pure saffron paste, mixed with a little bit of wax. Some women of her generation had a tiny spot tattooed on the center of their foreheads when they were still very young girls. This was to help them position their *tilak* perfectly. But most of us just made a well-practiced guess. We had lovely little silver boxes to keep our *kumkum*, the red powder used for our *tilaks* and some of us had a little trousseau of *kumkum* applicators, like keys on a chain. They looked like tiny little cookie cutters or branding irons on the end of tooth-picks, except that everything was wrought in silver. The shapes were so sweet: a little crescent moon, a star, or a tiny flower. We dipped these in the *kumkum* and pressed them to our foreheads. The powder remained like that throughout the day, because we first put a little spot of wax exactly where the *tilak* would sit.

Nowadays women use stick-on *tilaks*. I don't think my maids would allow me to do that; but I do cling to a little black *tilak* even though I am a widow. I love that little *tikka*; it's become part of me, and I don't think my husband would mind. He left such things to me. In fact, he never objected when long before his death, I stopped wearing *sindur* in the parting of my hair. In our time, *sindur* and the *tilak* were red *kumkum* powders, made by soaking turmeric rhizomes for a week in lemon juice and borax and then grinding them into a fine, red powder. In the old days, Hindu women wore *sindur* in the parting of the hair to indicate that they had attained that coveted status of *suhagan*, *soubhagya*, or marriage. Some people say it is also a symbol of a woman's modesty, covering even that tiny fraction of her anatomy from the gaze of anyone but her husband! But *sindur* was going out of fashion even in my day, though I find that in recent times there has been a revival of using *sindur*, thanks to the women in the plethora of television soaps who always wear it so proudly!

Kaajal, which is traditional, is still very much in use today. It must be made very carefully of the purest ingredients; then it really does benefit the eyes, besides making them more beautiful. I have already described my mother's method for making excellent *kaajal*; but in Madanpur we had a far more elaborate, romantic method. The whole process began on the night of the fullest full moon of the year. We call that moon Sharad Purnima. It falls in the season of Sharad, which is the months of October and November. We believe that on the night of Sharad Purnima, the gods send down *amrit*, or nectar, to the world through the rays of this most lovely full moon. Anything that is left to lie out in this full moon absorbs the goodness and auspiciousness of its rays and can pass that along to others.

In many princely states as well as private homes, all of the cooking utensils and vessels were put out in the kitchen courtyard on Sharad Purnima to absorb the moon's rays. This was not done willy-nilly; it was a solemn ceremony; like a play in fairyland and all of us were the actors. Everything, all the props in the play were of white, in honor of the occasion. The actual celebration took place on the shores of a lake not far from the palace compound. Cushions and bolsters of snow white silk were spread out for us to sit on, embroidered with silver thread and mirrors. *Zenana* women wore pearl colored clothes of satin and silk, which were also embroidered in silver. We wore no other jewelry but pearls: necklaces, earrings, bangles, and anklets of pearl glowed like the moon above us.

We laughed and danced until that moon disappeared; and we even had an auspicious picnic. Huge silver vessels filled with rice pudding, called *kheer*, were set out to absorb the moon's rays. We picnicked on this *kheer* and other dishes, all of them pure white.

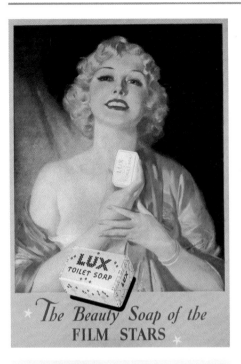

The Beauty Soap of the
FILM STARS

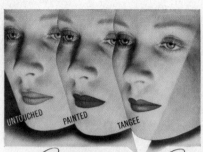

UNTOUCHED   PAINTED   TANGEE

Lip secrets of a Lady

This year lips of the smartest women are softly subdued—natural. The hard, coarse "painted look" is passé.

And this new vogue is the reason why Tangee is preferred by today's smartest women. For Tangee can't give you that "painted look" because *it isn't paint!* Instead Tangee changes color from orange in the stick to a lovely blush-rose on your lips. Blends with your own natural skin tones, and gives your lips a warm, feminine appeal.

Try Tangee. It stays on for hours and its special cream base keeps your lips soft and smooth. And when you buy . . . be sure to ask for Tangee Natural.

There is another shade of Tangee called Theatrical . . . but it is intended only for those who insist on vivid color, and for theatrical use. Tangee comes in three sizes . . . at all leading stores. Beware of substitutes when you buy. Don't let some sharp sales person switch you to an imitation...there's only one Tangee.

Other Famous Tangee Products

Tangee Face Powder now contains the magic Tangee color principle. Ends that "powdered" look. Tangee Rouge Compact blends with your own complexion. Tangee Creme Rouge is waterproof and protects the skin. All harmonize with Tangee Lipstick. Tangee Cosmetic darkens and beautifies your eyelashes and eyebrows. Does not irritate or run.

World's Most Famous Lipstick

TANGEE
ENDS THAT PAINTED LOOK

Sold by all chemists and stores throughout India,
Burma, Ceylon and Malaya.

Sales Agents : Muller Maclean & Co., Inc.

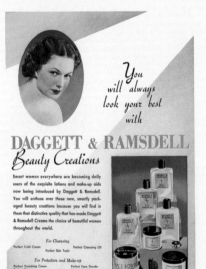

*You
will always
look your best
with*

DAGGETT & RAMSDELL
Beauty Creations

Smart women everywhere are becoming daily users of the exquisite lotions and make-up aids now being introduced by Daggett & Ramsdell. You will enthuse over these new, smartly packaged beauty creations because you will find in them that distinctive quality that has made Daggett & Ramsdell Creams the choice of beautiful women throughout the world.

For Cleansing
Perfect Cold Cream   Perfect Cleansing Oil
        Perfect Skin Tonic

For Protection and Make-up
Perfect Vanishing Cream   Perfect Face Powder
Perfect Rouge   Perfect Lipstick
Perfect Eyeshadow   Perfect Eyebrow Pencil

For the Hair   **For the Hands**
Perfect Oil Shampoo   Perfect Hand Lotion

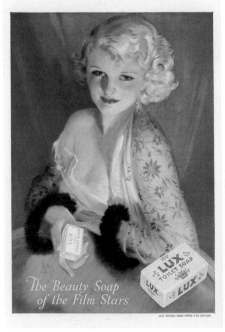

The Beauty Soap
of the Film Stars

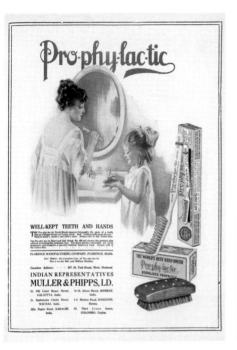

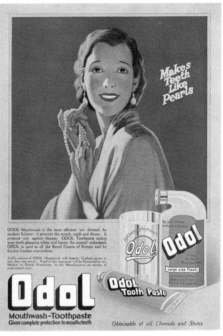

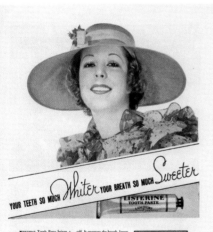

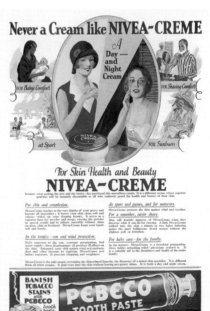

ff to one side of our sumptuous picnic sat big baskets of cotton wool. This nectar-filled cotton that had absorbed the moon's rays would be used to make the wicks for the lamps with which we would then make our *kaajal*. Fifteen days after Sharad Purnima comes Kali Chaudus or Roop Chaudus. Kali Chaudus is part of Diwali, our festival of lights, the biggest festival of the Hindu year. On that day we would take little tufts of that auspicious cotton and roll them tightly into wicks for the oil lamps. To the cotton we added powdered dill and bishop's weed or *ajwain* seeds for their medicinal properties. Then we burned those wicks in clarified butter or mustard oil to make our *kaajal* for the year.

We turned a little copper or silver cup over the flame to catch the soot, then collected this in a small silver box and mixed it with some clarified butter. That part was the same as my mother's method. But in Madanpur, there was an additional, more elaborate procedure, thanks to the good Pandit Dubey. He proclaimed that *kaajal* was not really beneficial unless it was kept for a few weeks in a Margosa *neem* tree, tucked into the hollow of a branch. Perhaps he recommended this because the *neem* is cooling? He never did enlighten me, but I know that the cooling aspect is important. So people went to even greater lengths than Pandit Dubey to render the *kaajal* cooling: they actually put it in a wooden box and immersed it in a river for at least six months. We never went that far. For the most part, these old, elaborate practices have disappeared; though women continue to make *kaajal* in the simple manner my mother used.

There was also something else we used to cool our eyes and add luster to them. That was a dry powder called *surma*. In our time *surma* was made from real seed pearls, which were processed into a silvery ash by those secret ayurvedic methods that Pandit Dubey practiced and would often tell me about.

Speaking of *surma* reminds me of another, rather beautiful adornment that the women of Hyderabad used. It was a very fine powder called *afshaan*. You could only get *afshaan* in a special *galli* or street of the Hyderabad bazaar where everything for brides and weddings was sold in rows of shops. *Afshaan* was made from pure silver. Brides and married women had the right to dust a bit of that silver powder on their cheekbones to give themselves a special sparkle. Some of the bolder ones sprinkled it in their hair; that gave a very magical touch.

Most of us, as I have said, were not allowed or inclined to use cosmetics as we know them today. Even in matters of hygiene, our recourse was always to things natural. We didn't use toothpaste to keep our teeth clean and bright; we used the twig of a tree from the garden, a *neem* tree, that same one into which we tucked our *kaajal* to imbibe its cooling properties. *Neem* twigs were cut fresh from the garden each morning and placed in the bathrooms by our maids. That was palace procedure but I know that in towns and villages everywhere, *neem* twigs are available even today—a fresh one every day for brushing, chewing, and massaging one's gums. *Neem* twigs are terribly bitter, but excellent both for cleaning the mouth and for sweetening the breath after eating.

The idea was to chew on the tip of the twig until its ends frayed to form a sort of natural brush. The bitter juice was to be spat out, not swallowed; still it was considered very beneficial. *Neem* was used in many different ways. I remember that on the day of the Hindu New Year, tender leaves and flowers of the *neem* were pounded and roasted with black pepper, cumin, and sugar in a little clarified butter. Everyone in the family had to eat a little of this mixture in the belief that it would cure all diseases. According to ayurvedic doctors, bitter foods are very good for one's health as they remove all sorts of poisons from the body, thereby purifying the blood.

Wherever *neem* was not available, people used twigs of other trees or else natural tooth powders. Some used tooth powder made of charcoal and salt; others used something called *geru mitti*, a special red earth mixed with ginger, long pepper, black pepper, cloves, camphor, and menthol. Still others brushed their teeth with roasted tobacco or plain salt. I personally have used a preparation of salt, pepper, alum, and almond skins that is excellent. The skins are burned over live coals, then powdered and sifted with a fine sieve. My granddaughter said her dentist recommended this very same remedy quite recently for her little daughter's sore gums!

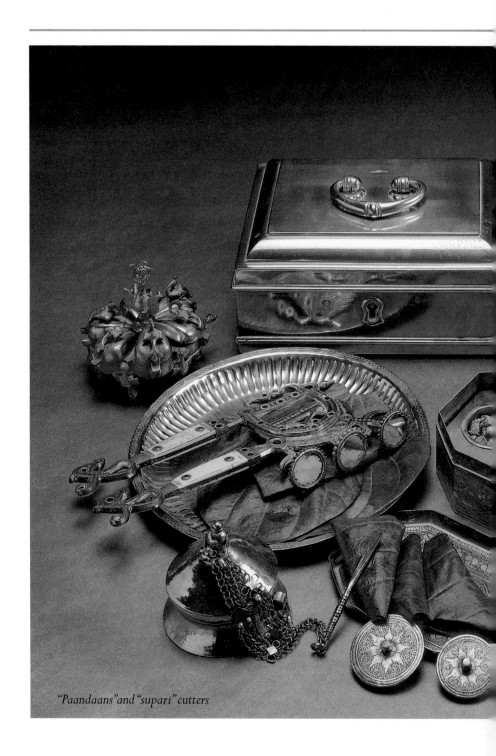

"Paandaans"and"supari" cutters

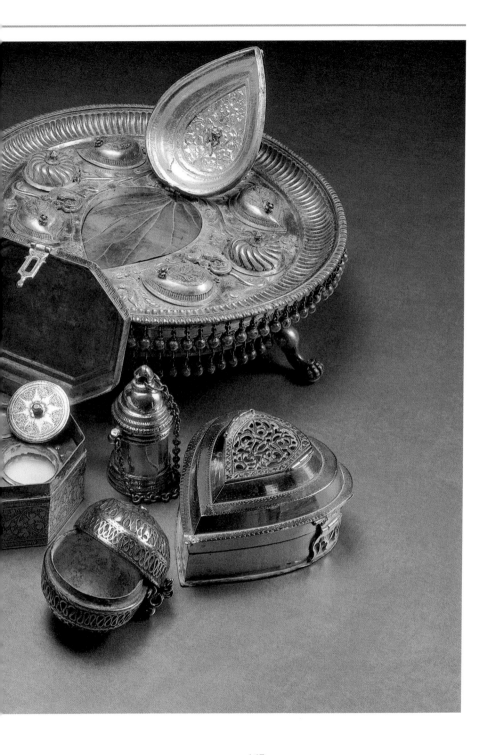

All these preparations are truly good for the teeth and gums; some of them sweeten the breath as well. But for that purpose our favorite was always the betel leaf, *paan*. *Paan* was our enduring passion in the *zenana* and I still cannot do without it. This was the one point upon which dear Miss Blake and I could not ever compromise politely. She found the chewing of *paan* disgusting, just as I found it absolutely delightful. Like all women in the *zenana*, I liked the red color it lent to my lips and the taste bordered on an addiction.

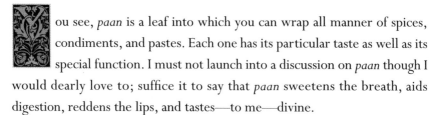ou see, *paan* is a leaf into which you can wrap all manner of spices, condiments, and pastes. Each one has its particular taste as well as its special function. I must not launch into a discussion on *paan* though I would dearly love to; suffice it to say that *paan* sweetens the breath, aids digestion, reddens the lips, and tastes—to me—divine.

Miss Blake did not approve of my *paan*-chewing at all; but she loved the little box in which I kept all the ingredients to put into that *paan*. She was fascinated by the ingredients themselves: yellow cardamom, golden saffron, black cloves, brown nutmeg, yellow-green anise, pearly white grated coconut, white slaked lime, and tan *catechu* pastes. The betel nut itself is small, hard, and brown; we call it *supari*. All these delicacies lay in their little containers nestled in my lovely chased silver *paan* box. In the center of the box were the shiny green betel leaves shaped like aces of hearts. We folded all those various ingredients into these leaves. The whole thing was an art and a solemn ritual; we took the eating and offering of *paan* very seriously in the palace.

Pandit Dubey used to say that the ingredients for *paan*, when taken together, were potent with thirteen qualities. He loved to enumerate them: bitterness, pungency, heat, sweetness, saltiness, and astringency, also the ability to eliminate gas and phlegm from the body, to stimulate the libido, and to render the mouth sweet, fresh, and pure. "The qualities to be found in *paan*," he used to sigh, "are unattainable anywhere else, even in heaven!" Many of us agree with him.

Paan is a very ancient habit and a lot of etiquette is involved. We have a saying, "a betel leaf presented with respect is a great gift." In other words the

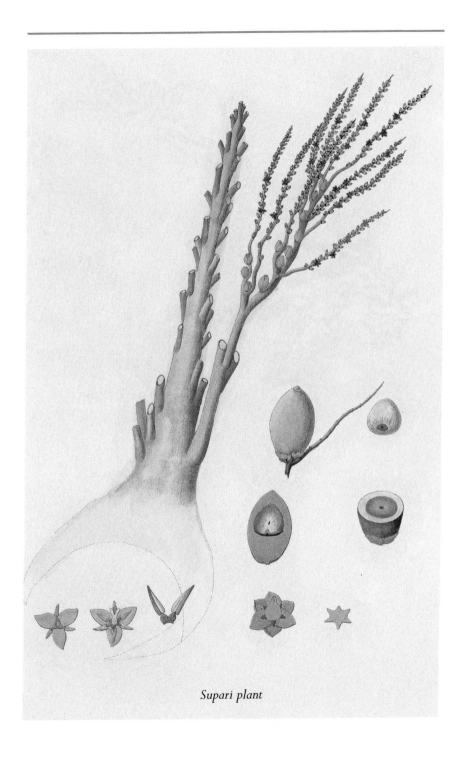

Supari plant

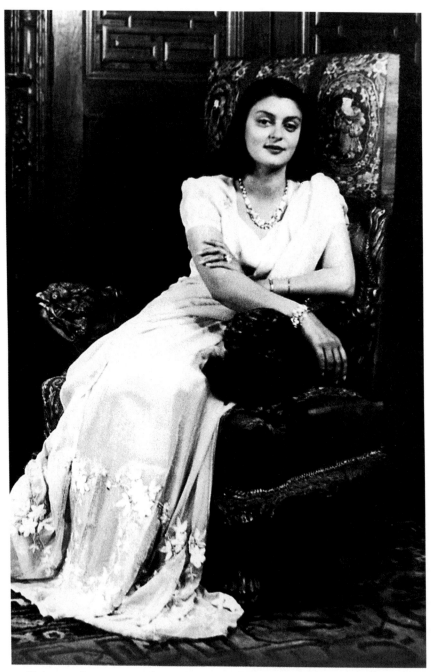

Maharani Gayatri Devi of Jaipur, one of the most beautiful women in the world

offering or exchanging of a *paan* leaf represented for us, in the old courtly circles, much more than just proffering something to share, like you would offer a cigarette to someone. The presentation of a *paan* could be imbued with different meanings: respect, hospitality, or even mutual trust—as when rulers of two different princely states each took a bite of the same *paan*, thus indicating that they were willing to share the risk of its being poisoned.

n festive occasions, it was the task of the *zenana* women to prepare the *paans* that were offered to the guests after the banquet. We had a lot of fun. We sat in a large circle, laughing, gossiping, and teasing each other as we worked. We washed the betel leaves, snipped off the stems, and laid out the leaves in rows. We piled on the various ingredients and finally folded them into different shapes: cones or triangles or little squares held together with a clove. In the old days even the way a *paan* leaf was folded could convey a message such as, "He's away, so I'm free tonight!" Such are the arts one can learn in a *zenana*!

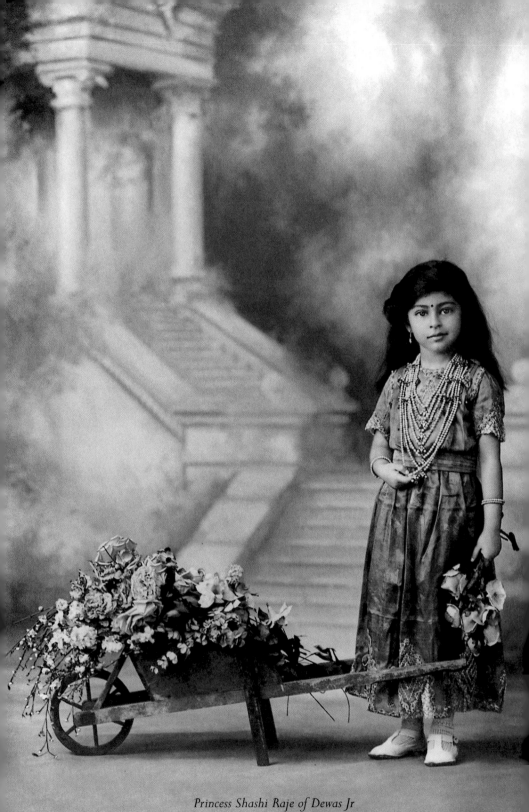

Princess Shashi Raje of Dewas Jr

9.

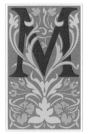

Myriad Fragrances

"Putting peacock feathers on a crow's tail!" That's what we say about futile vanity, about anyone as homely as that awful crow being vain enough to fuss with appearance! Well, here I am, for all the world like that crow, having my massage, using *utanas*, still dressing and oiling my hair. I still, good heavens, use perfume, though it's strictly off-limits for widows. Oh! But I love scent. It holds so many memories. Scent brings back my childhood, beloved friends, familiar garments, seasons, and above all, ceremonies.

Nothing can take that away; it's inside me. But if I summon it all back with scent now and then, I'm sure the gods will forgive me. I have only to open a bottle and I'm away into another era.

There is essence of sandalwood, for example; one of my earliest pleasures is that fragrance. For me sandalwood meant coolness, purity, and a very special peace. I used to sit with my mother in her *puja* room, the room where she worshipped her gods, and I would rub the sandalwood to a paste for her, sitting on the floor of that dimly lit room with the coolness of stone on my legs. I would take a little stick of pure sandalwood and rub it round and round on a small marble slab. Slowly it yielded itself into a paste, coaxed by drops of water. That paste was so soft: we only needed a tablespoon for the daily *puja*.

My mother would daub some on the forehead of each of the gods after she had bathed them in milk. You see in India, Hindu deities have their beauty rituals just as we human beings do, using the very same ingredients: turmeric, *kumkum* powder, honey, milk, yogurt, *ritha*, clarified butter, oil, saffron, camphor, sandalwood, flowers, incense, and perfume! My mother's deities were of silver, small as a paperweight, older than anyone remembered. Every morning my mother would wash each of them in water and *ritha*, the very same soapnuts we used for bathing. Then she would dry them with a little piece of muslin and dress them in garments she had made of brocade. Every year at Diwali, our festival of lights, the gods got new garments just as we did. They also had minute little ornaments made of gold and precious stones. Mother would arrange all this carefully every day before applying the sandalwood paste, saffron, *kumkum,* and turmeric with the ring finger of her right hand.

On the head of each little god, she would then place a freshly plucked blossom, usually a jasmine or a marigold. I can see her still, her head covered by the fall of her *odhna*; her face lit by the glow of the little oil lamp she used to perform her *aarti*. She always sang softly while she did the *aarti*, passing the tray of light gently round the gods, asking for and returning their blessing.

Everything used for *puja* had to be very, very, pure—undefiled by any action or presence that might be disrespectful. I had difficulty sometimes restraining myself in accordance with these dictates of purity, for I loved to smell that sandalwood as I rubbed it into a paste. Whenever I thought my mother wasn't looking, I would quickly lift my fingers to my nose and inhale its delicate, spicy aroma. I was not supposed to do that or, for that matter, to smell the flowers that were laid out as an offering to the gods.

But fortunately, on other occasions, sandalwood paste was permitted to us children. I almost enjoyed having prickly heat, because the remedy was sandalwood paste. To this day that fragrance takes me back to the coolness and peace of my mother's *puja* room, which was truly a sanctuary. The very thought of coolness has an attraction for us in India that others may not understand. We long for it and seek refuge in it just as people who live in cold climates seek solace round a cozy fireplace. I never realized this until I went to Kashmir with Miss Blake just before my marriage. It was my first experience of genuine cold. Then I understood that our winters in Rajasthan were not really cold, just pleasantly chilly.

The nuance of our seasons is so different from that of other places in the world. We know nothing of the summer, winter, autumn, and spring Miss Blake described to me so often. Our seasons are spring, summer, monsoons, and chill. Spring is hot and full of flowers, but still the heat is bearable. By summer, everyone's preoccupation is simply surviving until the rains. When the monsoons come, the skies cloud if we are lucky, and the rains fall in spells for three months or more. Monsoons are a blessed relief from the heat. They lead us into our winter, a mere two or three months of the year when we can shiver a bit and burrow down into big quilts.

It is not a real winter, according to Miss Blake, but for us each of those seasons has its special joys. Also, each has its perfume. I shall begin with winter perfumes. The thought of that cold brings to mind one of my favorite memories: the heavy quilts we used in that season. Those quilts, which we called *razais,* were filled with cotton and actually sprayed with "heating" essences by means of a tiny syringe. We used the potent *agar* and musk essences for our quilts; I shall speak of them later. We also used the same amber which we blushingly daubed between our breasts when we thought that the aunties weren't looking. Then there was *hina* distilled from the very same henna that we used to highlight our hair and to stain pretty patterns on our palms. In winter we wore those perfumes on our bodies, applied very discreetly of course, and we also slept snuggled in quilts that smelled of them.

When spring came in March, or really mid-February, we changed to lighter quilts that we used right into summer. These were very thin, just a covering really. They were injected with "cooling" essences like the rose essence and *khus* made from vetiver root, the same *khus* that was woven into matting hung on the doors and windows and sprayed with water for cooling our rooms. Again, we also wore these same cooling fragrances on our bodies as perfumes, or as we called them, *attars* or *ittrs.*

When spring came, all the winter clothes and quilts had to be stored in big chests. First everything was washed and aired for a few days, spread all

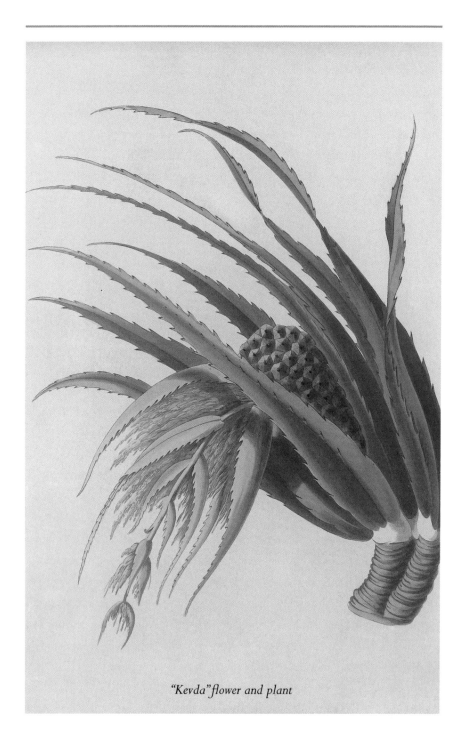

"Kevda" flower and plant

over the courtyard in an absolute riot of color. The maids would bring baskets of dried *neem* leaves. Bless that *neem* tree! It's good for so many things: from soothing skin rashes to purifying the blood, to keeping insects out of clothes. A cushion of *neem* leaves lined the bottom of each chest, then came the layers of clothes. Each garment was individually wrapped in folds of muslin with a sprinkling of black pepper and cloves. The pepper and cloves were extra insurance against insects. To this day I use them: their pungent, spicy aroma is so much more pleasant than the smell of those naphthalene balls. I never use naphthalene, not even for carpets, which I always roll up for the two or three months of monsoon. Instead, I sprinkle them with dried tobacco leaves and I've never yet had a moth hole.

Combating insects has become a sort of art in India; we have to deal with so many of them. In the old days solutions to the insect problem were really very aesthetic as well as effective. I remember, for instance, the way we packed those wonderful quilts to preserve them from the bugs. They were first smoked, just like we smoked our hair after a bath. But this smoking was really fumigation against insects. *Agar* was the best incense for that purpose, the very same *agar* that was said to be potent in a *paan*! But I shall come to that shortly.

When I think back on those days in the palace, I realize our whole existence was filled with fragrance. Apart from seasonal scents, there were the fragrances that became very dear and very much a part of our lives. There were the fragrant flowers plucked each morning and woven into garlands for our hair and for the *puja*. There were the scents of the *puja* room: sandalwood, camphor, and incense.

Then every evening there was a very special smell as the household lamps were lit. This lamp lighting happened in every home, not just in palaces. In Madanpur, it was done with an enormous oil torch called a *mashaal*, but in other homes, small lamps of silver, brass, or even clay would be lit. Even in a palace, it was always the duty of the daughters-in-law to light the lamps at twilight. First the little tray of light was taken to their mother- and father-in-law and presented for their blessings. In turn, each daughter-in-law would touch the feet of the elders and accept their blessings on her head.

W hen the first lamp in the household was lit, everyone, family and servants alike, would say a fleeting little prayer and fold their hands for a moment. That moment is sacred to Hindus. We think of the sun as synonymous with God. So when the sun goes down, the light replacing it is also sacred. We have a saying: "The house where the elders are not heeded, the lamp is not lit, and the wife is barren, will be ruined."

I am happy to say that I remember Madanpur during the days when all those conditions were fulfilled and our household was richly content. The fragrance of that contentment shall always be for me the fragrance of an incense called *dhup* or *loban*, for at the same time as the lamps were lit every evening, this incense was carried from room to room in a beautiful silver censer. The sweet smoke from the censer hung in each room like a silent visitor. I never thought of *dhup* as an insect repellent, but it did serve to keep them away. In my father's palace, the incense came from a town called Ashapura where a whole mountain of *dhup* was found.

Miss Blake said *dhup* was the very same frankincense that the Wise Men brought to baby Jesus. We used to wonder about this, because the Wise Men's gifts of gold, frankincense, and myrrh are all highly valued and much used in India. Gold has always been considered to have wonderful healing properties according to ayurveda. Myrrh too, has been used here as medicine since prehistoric times. We call this fragrant resin *hirabol* or *guggal* and use it as a remedy for a number of children's aliments.

Winter, that bracing season when we could snuggle under quilts and wear our heaviest silks, was over far too quickly. The festival of Holi, in the middle of March, marked the beginning of spring. At Holi, we always had one last burst of outdoor activity, a real orgy, not of wine, but of color. Everyone threw colored powder on each other and squirted one another with colored water from ingenious silver syringes. All this took

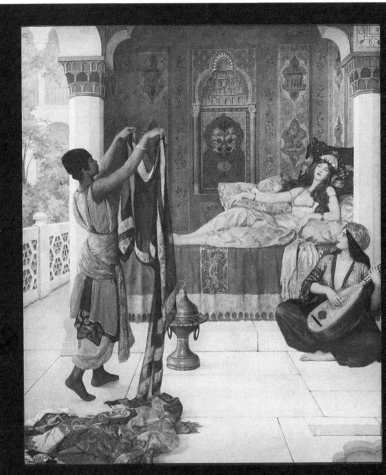

MYRRH, ALOES & CASSIA.
BY THE HON. JOHN COLLIER.

"ERASMIC"
Soaps & Perfumes.
Luxurious and Delightful.

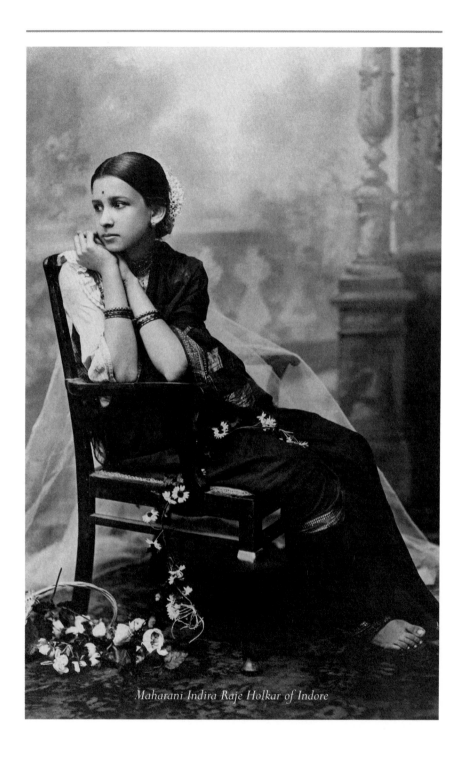

Maharani Indira Raje Holkar of Indore

place against a background of the most brilliant flowers. Everything in nature blossoms in spring and our garments were no match for the garden in that season.

ut very soon after Holi, the heat made its presence felt. After that it was possible to pretend you were cold, only by sitting in a room whose windows were covered in thick woven matting made from the roots of a desert plant we know as *khus*, which Miss Blake called vetiver. *Khus* emitted the most heavenly, indescribable fragrant coolness when it was dampened and kept in a breeze. Its smell was the smell of coolness itself; I know no other way to describe it.

We even added a bit of that *khus* to the huge earthen pots that cooled our drinking water in the summer. Sometimes we put a few fresh jasmine flowers into that water. Throughout summer we quenched our thirst with a special cooling drink made with almonds: take five almonds and soak them overnight in cold water. In the morning, remove the skins and grind them with a little sugar candy. We used to dilute this with the fragrant *khus* water and drink it throughout the day.

The "magicians" who make our myriad scents in India know how to distill seasons and moods into an essence. *Khus* is a perfume, or rather an essence, that can be bought in a bottle. But to me it brings back the very same coolness and contentment I felt sitting by that *khus* matting. All over India one can buy essences we refer to as *attars*. *Attars* cover the gamut of possible fragrance, from cool like *khus* and sandalwood to earthy, like *mitti*. *Mitti attar* has the smell of fields in the first showers of the much longed for monsoons. *Attars* can also smell of flowers; there are wonderful floral fragrances, most of which we used in spring and summer.

My father-in-law was a great connoisseur of these. He had beautiful boxes like humidors, fitted out with shelves and exquisite bottles, each with a special stopper. His *attars* were carefully arranged according to their formulations. The florals were grouped together: there was rose, *kamal* or lotus, *kevda, champa,* and *raat rani*—Queen of the Night—a tiny white flower with a heavy perfume that flowers only when the sun goes down. Then there were all the jasmines: *mogra*, *chameli*, *motia*, and *juhi,* Each of them were to be used with the greatest discretion; a little goes a long way.

I suppose that is why the bottles were no bigger than a test tube. Even essences made from the fragrant grasses were kept in very small bottles. My father-in-law had a preference for these essences: *khus* or vetiver, lemon and blue grass, citrus grass and *rusa*; also essence made from the leaves of henna and *marwa*. He used to put them on his body or his garments or carry a scented hanky. In the beginning, of course, this puzzled Miss Blake. She had never known men to wear scent in this way. It was something she had always associated with women. I always suspected that she continued to do so, though I explained many times that in our culture, both sexes enjoyed perfumes.

shared my father-in-law's love for scent and also kept boxes full of bottles. But I know that many people cannot afford that. The merchant who supplied us with scent at the palace told me that people in the bazaar go about the matter of perfume in a manner that leaves them a great deal of choice, but requires no investment at all. They merely stroll down to the perfumer's shop and buy a *faya* for a few paise. A *faya* is a little cotton bud rolled at the end of a long stick and dipped into the selected essence. The customer removes the perfumed bud, tucks it into the little fold at the top of his ear and wipes the excess onto his clothes and body. Women also buy such *fayas* to tuck into their cupboards and clothes.

How I loved my bottles of perfume! Wherever I went, I made it a point to seek out the *attars* of that region and add them to my collection. Usually they came complete with a story, as for example, *attar* of roses. There is a very romantic story attached to that fragrance. I have heard it in many versions. But the essence of the story concerns an empress of the Mughal court, the fabulous seventeenth-century court of the Muslims who ruled India for three hundred years from their capital in Delhi. It is said that *attar* of roses was discovered by the beautiful Nur Jahan at the time of her marriage to

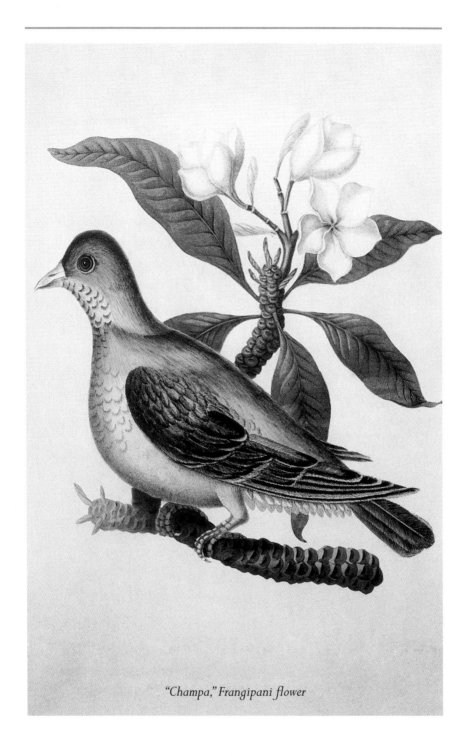

"Champa," Frangipani *flower*

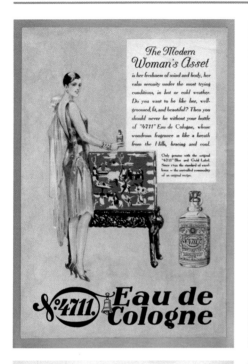

The Modern
Woman's Asset

is her freshness of mind and body, her
calm serenity under the most trying
conditions, in hot or cold weather.
Do you want to be like her, well-
groomed, fit, and beautiful? Then you
should never be without your bottle
of "4711" Eau de Cologne, whose
wondrous fragrance is like a breath
from the Hills, bracing and cool.

Only genuine with the original
"4711" Blue and Gold Label.
Since 1792 the standard of excel-
lence — the unrivalled commodity
of an original recipe.

№ 4711 Eau de Cologne

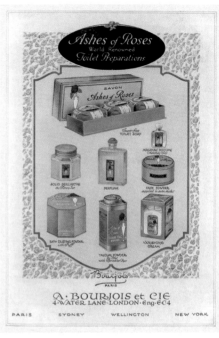

Ashes of Roses
World Renowned
Toilet Preparations

A. BOURJOIS et CIE
4 WATER LANE · LONDON · Eng · EC4

PARIS   SYDNEY   WELLINGTON   NEW YORK

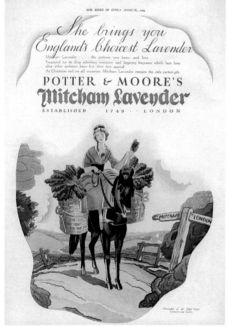

She brings you
England's Choicest Lavender

Mitcham Lavender . . . . the perfume you know and love . . . .
Treasured for its deep refreshing sweetness and lingering fragrance which lasts long
after other perfumes have lost their first appeal.
At Christmas and on all occasions Mitcham Lavender remains the only perfect gift.

POTTER & MOORE'S
Mitcham Lavender

ESTABLISHED · 1749 · · LONDON

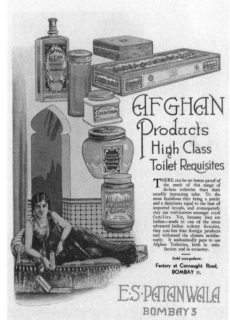

AFGHAN
Products
High Class
Toilet Requisites

THERE can be no better proof of
the merit of this range of
de-luxe toiletries than their
steadily increasing sales. To the
most fastidious they bring a purity
and a daintiness equal to the best of
imported brands, and consequently
they are well-known amongst royal
families. Yet, because they are
Indian—made in one of the most
advanced Indian toiletry factories,
they cost less than foreign products
and withstand the climate satisfac-
torily. It undoubtedly pays to use
Afghan Toiletries, both in satisfaction and in economy.

Sold everywhere.

Factory at Connaught Road,
BOMBAY 11.

E·S·PATANWALA
BOMBAY 3

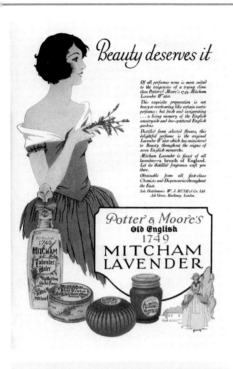

Beauty deserves it

Of all perfumes none is more suited to the exigencies of a trying clime than Potter & Moore's 1749 Mitcham Lavender Water.

This exquisite preparation is not heavy or overbearing like certain exotic perfumes; but fresh and invigorating ... a living memory of the English countryside and dew-spattered English gardens.

Distilled from selected flowers, this delightful perfume is the original Lavender Water which has ministered to Beauty throughout the reigns of seven English monarchs.

Mitcham Lavender is finest of all lavenders—a breath of England. Let its distilled fragrance waft you there.

Obtainable from all first-class Chemists and Depôts everywhere in the East.

Sole Distributors: W. J. BUSH & Co. Ltd.
Ash Grove, Hackney, London.

Potter & Moore's Old English 1749 MITCHAM LAVENDER

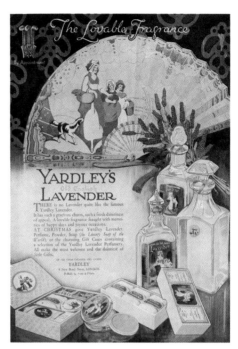

The Lovable Fragrance

By Appointment

YARDLEY'S Old English LAVENDER

THERE is no Lavender quite like the famous Yardley Lavender. It has such a gracious charm, such a fresh distinctness of appeal. A lovable fragrance fraught with memories of happy days and joyous occasions.

AT CHRISTMAS give Yardley Lavender: Perfume, Powder, Soap (the Luxury Soap of the World); or the charming Gift Cases containing a selection of the Yardley Lavender Perfumes. All make the most welcome and the daintiest of little Gifts.

OF ALL GOOD CHEMISTS AND STORES
YARDLEY
8 New Bond Street, LONDON

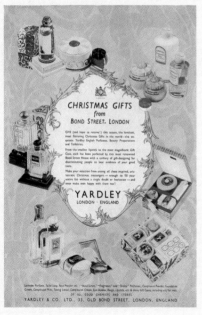

CHRISTMAS GIFTS from BOND STREET, LONDON

GIVE (and hope to receive!) this season, the loveliest, most flattering Christmas Gifts in the world—the exquisite Yardley English Perfumes, Beauty Preparations and Toiletries.

From the smallest lipstick to the most magnificent Gift Case, each has been perfected by this most renowned Bond Street House with a century of gift-designing for discriminating people to bear evidence of your good taste.

Make your selection from among all these inspired, aristocratic Christmas messengers—enough to fill your entire list without a single doubt or hesitation—and even make men happy with them too!

YARDLEY
LONDON · ENGLAND

YARDLEY & CO. LTD., 33, OLD BOND STREET, LONDON, ENGLAND

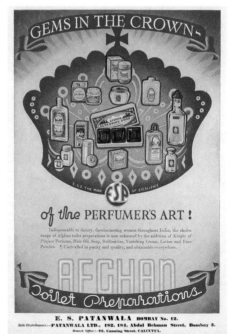

GEMS IN THE CROWN

of the PERFUMER'S ART !

Indispensable to dainty, discriminating women throughout India, the choice range of Afghan toilet preparations is now enhanced by the addition of Knight of Pinjore Perfume, Hair Oil, Soap, Brilliantine, Vanishing Cream, Lotion and Face Powder. ¶ Unrivalled in purity and quality, and obtainable everywhere.

AFGHAN Toilet Preparations

E. S. PATANWALA BOMBAY No. 12.
Sole Distributors:—PATANWALA LTD., 182, 184, Abdul Rehman Street, Bombay 3.
Branch Office :—72, Canning Street, CALCUTTA.

Emperor Jehangir, himself a great romantic. He had all the waterways in the palace filled with rose petals for the wedding. Nur Jahan noticed the oil that floated up from the blossoms and rested on the water's surface. She had it collected and found it to have a most bewitching fragrance, so she named it after her new husband: Attar-i-Jehangir.

ttar is, in fact, an Arabic word. Originally it was *ittr*, then the British anglicized it to *otto*. Otto came to mean the essence of roses in popular usage, but the Sanskrit word, before the Mughal invasion, was *saugandh*. Very few people would know that today. As with so many terms in our multilingual country, the Mughal word has predominated.

Mughals loved scent. Jehangir's father, the Emperor Akbar, perhaps the most glorious Mughal of them all, kept a special department devoted to perfumes. "His Majesty is very fond of perfumes and encourages the department from religious motives," records his chronicler, Ab'ul Fazl. "The court hall is continually scented with ambergris, aloe wood, and compositions according to ancient recipes or mixtures invented by His Majesty. Incense is daily burnt in gold and silver censers of various shapes; whilst sweet-smelling flowers are used in large quantities. Oils are extracted from flowers, and used for the skin and hair." In his case, there was no question of putting peacock feathers on a crow's tail; Akbar and his descendents were grand indeed.

But they had no monopoly on essences; historically Hindus have also had their fair share of fragrant indulgence, some of it rather exotic. My own father-in-law once showed me a box of exotic essence, quite separate from the pure fragrant ones. Pandit Dubey was witness to this and he explained some of the very strange things I saw in those bottles of oil. There was fat and entrails of tiger and bear, among other things. We passed over those rather rapidly and without explanation; but later in the bathing rooms I learned they were used for increasing what we blushingly called male potency.

The same was true for a fragrance called musk. His Highness had a real musk pod which the Pandit could not refrain from admiring. He said it comes from a gland in the stomach of the tiny musk deer which lives in the

Himalayas. We call the musk *kasturi*. It is extremely potent, as is another so-called aphrodisiac called *agar*, which is the resin obtained from the eagle-wood tree found only in East India.

Agar is a very strange scent. When applied to your body, it smells very unpleasant; but within half an hour, it alters somehow and begins to exude the most heavenly fragrance that when sniffed in its pure form, causes the nose to bleed. Pandit Dubey did not tell me this, but the *zenana* women swore there was a very famous *paan*, known as *palang-tod*, that contained minute quantities of either *kasturi* or *agar*.

Palang-tod means bed-breaker. I have never before told anyone that, but now that I have come out and said it, you know there was more than a bit of truth to all those stories of Indian aphrodisiacs. For better or for worse, we are left with nothing but a memory of musk and *agar* and hope for a brighter future. Once I advised a friend to use amber, and I actually gave her some of mine. Amber is found in the intestines of the sperm whale, according to the excellent Pandit. It is found floating on the sea and is very precious, as are other secretions from animals, like *zabad*, *gaura,* and *mid* which are derived from different species of the civet cat.

All of these essences are fraught with danger; or so our aunts would have us believe: "Just a little dab at your ears and wrists; if you're married, then a bit near your breasts!" I can hear them to this day, although I can assure you, in those days we hardly knew what they feared. We also diluted our essences so much that they scarcely provoked a reaction. *Attars* are strong. Miss Blake didn't like them, nor does my granddaughter. But I have always told them both, you must add alcohol to *attar* essences, then use them with great discretion.

On the other hand, courtesans, the dancers who used to come to the palace, wore very heavy perfume. I used to envy them that as well as their jewelry, not to mention their clothes. "Eat to please yourself, dress to please the world" is what we were told. So of course my dress, like my fragrant essences, was always modest in the extreme. But at those durbars, when the dancing girls appeared, I did allow myself to daydream a bit.

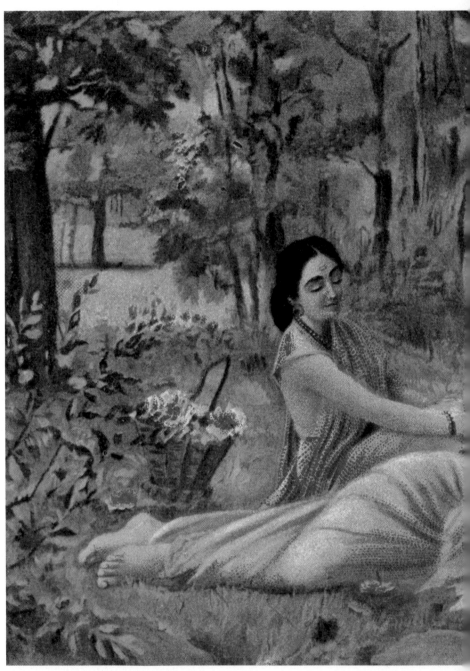

Enjoying the fragrance of the outdoors

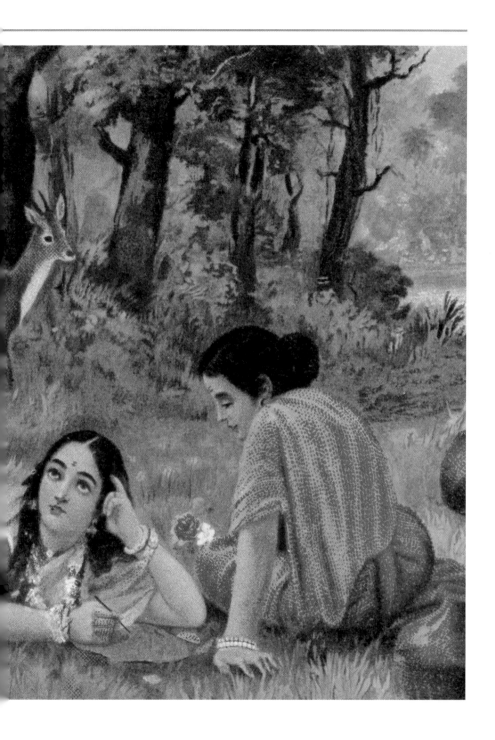

Dancing women and durbars remind me of another, entirely different fragrance, the sweetness of *attar* and *paan*. *Attar-paan* was a ceremony performed at those palace durbars, but also performed whenever a host wished to welcome his guest formally. *Attar*, as I have said, means perfumed essence. *Paan* was the leaf of the betel nut wrapped around various spices and condiments. But this *paan* had a very different meaning.

We say that "a *paan* presented with respect is as great a gift as a diamond." So we offer *paan* to a guest as a traditional gesture of hospitality and we also offer *attar*. The *attar* is usually kept in a small silver container to which a tiny spatula is attached. Using this spatula, the host daubs a bit of *attar* on the back of his guest's hand. It is always put on the hand, because then the wearer can discreetly and gracefully inhale the *attar* whenever the desire should strike him. This gesture of putting the back of the hand to the nose has traditionally been affected by haughty gentry putting on airs, like Europeans used to sniff their hankies. Be that as it may, I always found the *attar-paan* ritual charming, especially when the host or hostess sprinkled rose water, which we call *gulab-jal*, from a beautiful silver or gold container. It was done gracefully, from a little nozzle in the spout of the rose-water holder, often in the shape of a flower. Sometimes, as at our official durbars, it was sprinkled on the guest's outstretched hanky.

Rose will always remind me of durbars, just as sandalwood reminds me of *puja,* and *khus* reminds me of the very hot season. Perhaps nothing makes a stronger impression on our memories than the seasons we experience each year. Until recently there was very little to distance us from the rigors and the pleasures of those seasons. Now we can make artificial climate with air conditioning and heating and such. But in my best memories,there was no such imposition on our senses; we experienced our seasons, strong and pure.

One of our renowned poets, the famous Kalidasa, who lived in the fourth century, has written a poem on the seasons called *Ritusamhara*, "Garland of the Seasons," which expresses the rhythm and the joy of our seasons, passing from the heat to the cool of the monsoons, from the rains to the

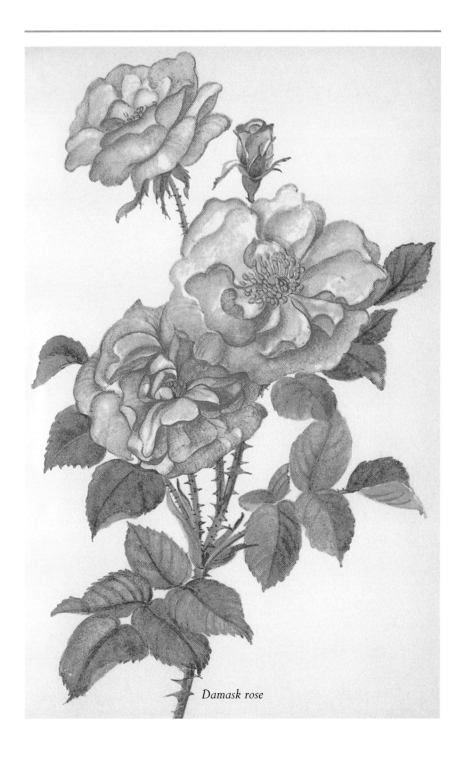

Damask rose

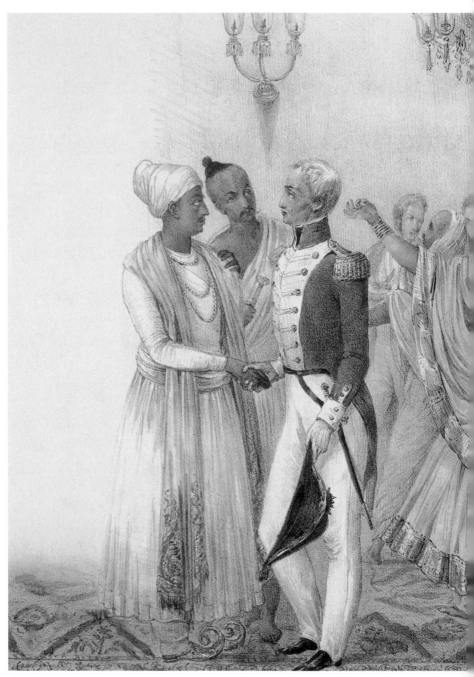

Courtesan entertaining guests

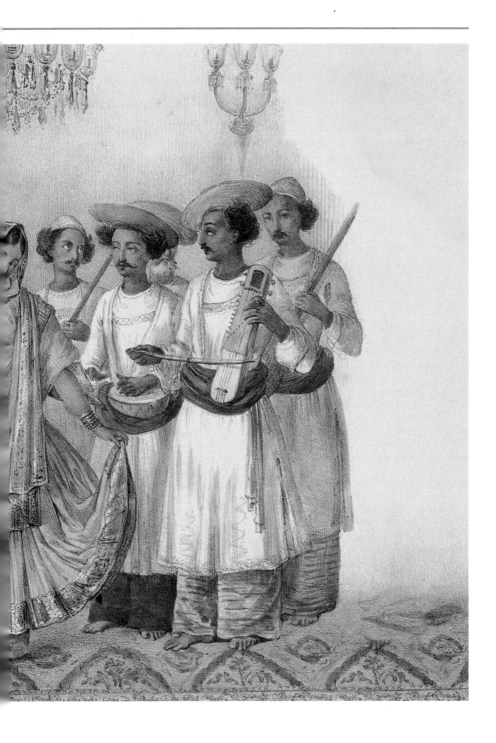

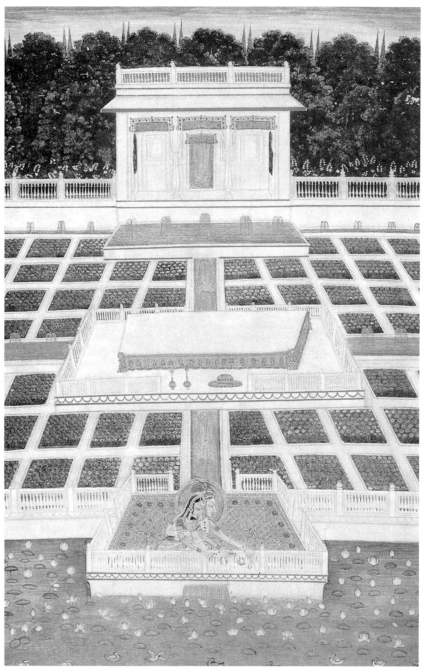

Lake of lotus blossoms

blessings of winter. He describes it all through lovely courtesans. Robed in transparent muslin in the heat of summer, they smear their breasts with sandal paste and their hair with light perfumes. Wearing flower garlands around their necks, they fan themselves with fans moistened in sandalwood water and swim in cool lakes full of lotus blossoms. Lac dye shines on the soles of their feet and jewels cold to the touch adorn their bodies.

uring the rains, the girls dress their hair with seasonal flowers and paint their bodies with the paste of eaglewood and sandalwood, to the accompaniment of rolls of thunder and flashes of lightning. Then comes autumn, when the trees are laden with flowers and the peacocks dance. The courtesans deck their bodies with jewelry and sandal paste and decorate their hair with lotus and jasmine blossoms. Winter is the time for women to paint their bodies with saffron paste, to wear pearl necklaces, and perfume their hair and bodies with musk. In late winter, when moonlit nights are no help to lovers, bedrooms are fumigated with the scent of musk. The women are bedecked with jewels and robes of soft silk. Then it's spring, the season for saffron colored and lac-dyed clothes, fumigated with black eaglewood.

I remember that my husband and I laughed at this very poem on our wedding night; he searching for his name in the palm of my hand; I undoing all the knots in his drawstring. How full of laughter and tears are these little things: as subtle as scent or the tinkle of an anklet; as bright as the colors of a wedding *sari*.

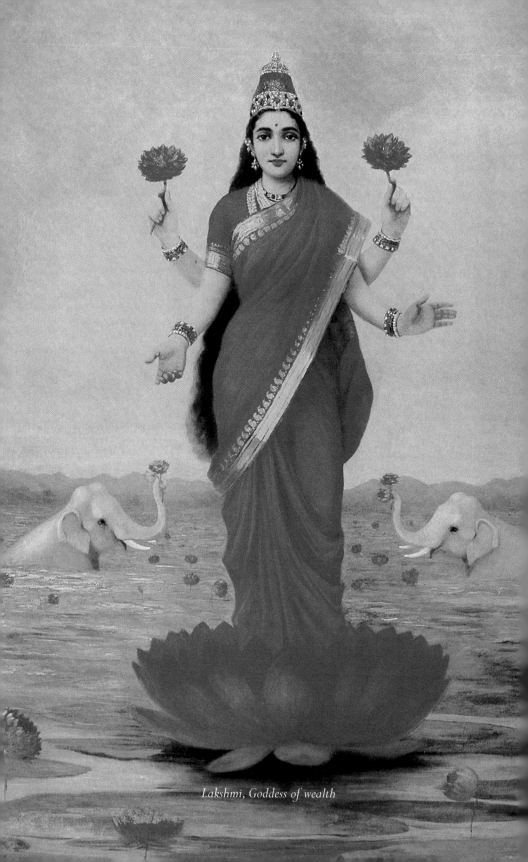

Lakshmi, Goddess of wealth

10.

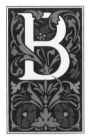

ejeweled and Bedecked

I am nearing the end of my book. At the very beginning I spoke of my people, the Rajputs of Rajasthan, and how much their honor mattered to them. All that seems so remote now, almost unbelievable; but I have known that life of chivalry, of pageantry and princes—or at least the tail end of it. I have felt the surge of pride in being Rajput royalty, just as I have chafed under all the restrictions that such a life imposes on women.

Over and over again I have repeated in this book that a woman in India is more than a woman, she is the symbol of her family's honor and well-being. She is Lakshmi, the goddess of wealth and prosperity; she must behave herself and adorn herself in a manner befitting that status. For royal women such as I was, this was doubly true, even though by the time I was born, it was already the twilight of an era.

I have spoken of *shringara*, our many beauty rituals; and of *saleekha*, our belief in moderate, balanced behavior, tempered by humility and respect. I have even spoken of matters I have never before dared mention in public like superstitions and marital relations. There remains still the matter of jewelry, the passion of both Indian men and women.

Jewelry for us is more than mere ornamentation; it is a proclamation of our prosperity and a reflection of our status. It is a source of beneficial qualities through the properties of the metals and stones, and a sort of mediator between ourselves and our fate, through the influence of the stones on our personal planets and their supposed intervention to protect us. For Indian women, jewelry is *stree-dhan*, a woman's wealth, gifted to her not only for adorning herself, but also as her security in times of need.

As a woman, princess, and symbolic Lakshmi, I was supposed to wear jewelry at all times, from my earliest childhood. Like so many children in India, my ears were pierced when I was still a baby. We in Rajasthan believe that a girl child achieves her own identity on the sixth day after her birth. On that day she becomes separate from her mother. So it was on that day that my ears were pierced and pure gold wires were threaded through them. That was my very first jewelry.

As I have said, we feel that gold is auspicious and beneficial. When I became a little older, a little ring of gold thread was pierced through my left nostril, where some day I would wear ornaments. I was also given golden ankle bracelets that jingled whenever I moved. The wearing of gold on one's feet was a privilege royalty reserved for itself; other women wore only silver. Later I was given much heavier anklets to steady my gait as I first walked.

Like so many other children, and adults for that matter, I wore a necklace around my neck at all times. There were two or three reasons for that. First, we believe that the gold in the necklace lends its goodness to the bathwater poured over it and this goodness washes over the body.

Second, the older women all insisted that wearing a necklace kept the neck very graceful; the heavier the necklace, the more slender the neck, was the old way of thinking. Later in life, women were supposed to wear a necklace to remind them that their heads must be bowed in humility.

The third reason for wearing a necklace had to do with superstition, or, if you like, the science of astrology. When I was born, my horoscope was cast. Based on that horoscope, the family astrologer recommended that I should wear certain stones and avoid others if my life was to be blessed by fortune. So as a tiny toddler, I wore a beautiful emerald on a heavy gold chain, because our *Raj Vaid* declared that emeralds would protect me and bring me happiness.

Many, many Indians strongly believe that wearing certain stones suits them and wearing others does not. They will seldom buy or wear a stone without first consulting their own astrologer or *vaid*. He will check the vari-

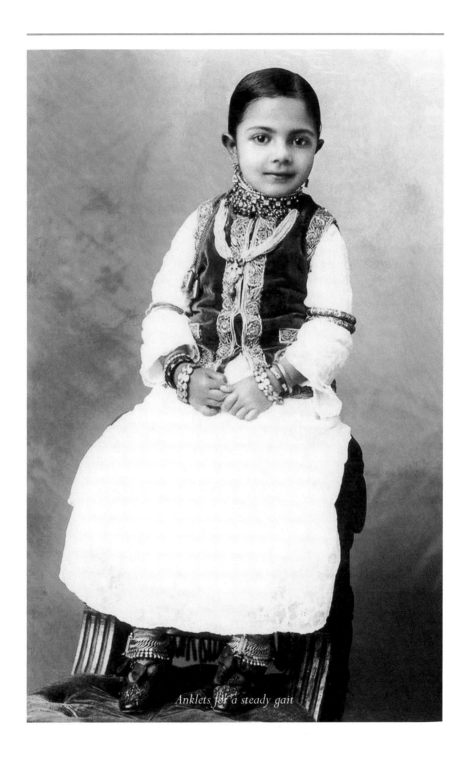

Anklets for a steady gait

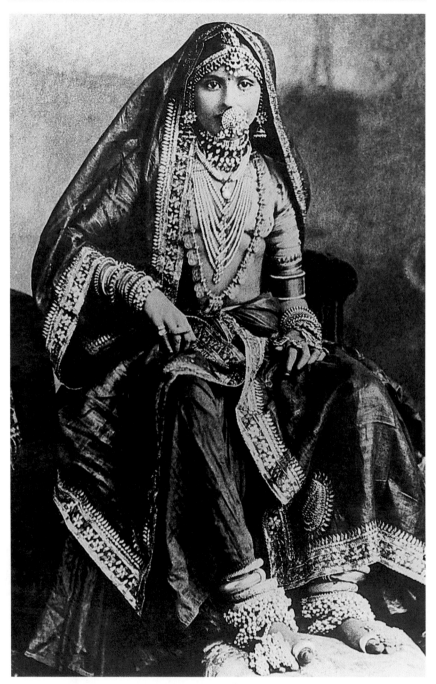

The burden of jewelry

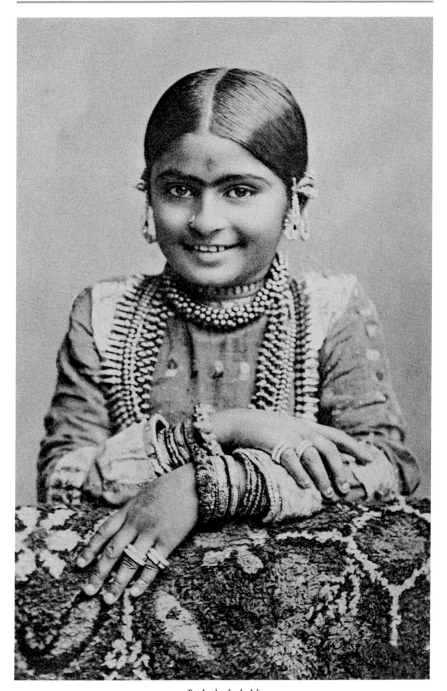

Bedecked child

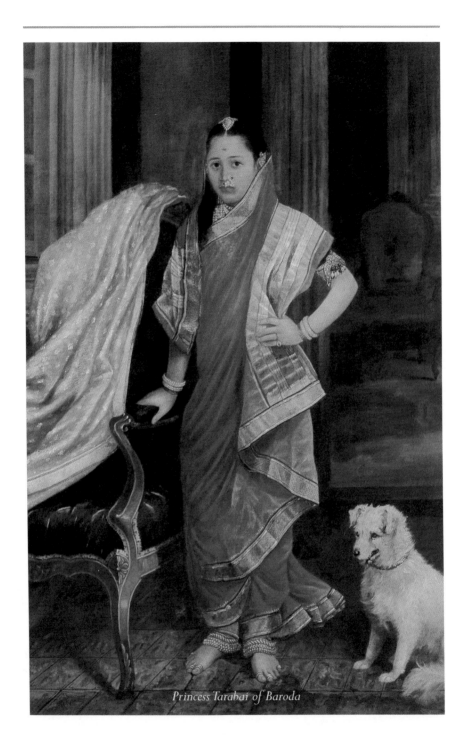

Princess Tarabai of Baroda

ous properties of that stone to see how they tally with the purchaser's horoscope and nature. Some stones, according to us, are simply not good for some people.

So jewelers are quite accustomed to giving a gem on approval. The client will wear it for a week and observe its effects. Some of them will soak the stone in milk, sleep with it under their pillow, and see how that affects their dreams. Certain stones are especially suspect—the blue sapphire in particular. We believe that blue sapphires suit very few people. In fact, few women dare to wear them.

His Highness the Maharaja of Madanpur's sister was widowed only six months after her marriage. The whole *zenana* blamed her fate on a blue sapphire one of the princes presented at her wedding. We knew she had never bothered to test its effect on her dreams, but had worn it straight away out of vanity and pride.

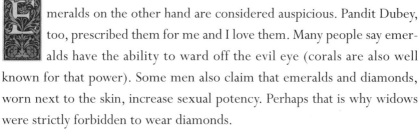meralds on the other hand are considered auspicious. Pandit Dubey, too, prescribed them for me and I love them. Many people say emeralds have the ability to ward off the evil eye (corals are also well known for that power). Some men also claim that emeralds and diamonds, worn next to the skin, increase sexual potency. Perhaps that is why widows were strictly forbidden to wear diamonds.

Goodness knows how much truth there is in all this. I do remember, however, that Pandit Dubey once recommended soaking an emerald in the water of a flower called *kevda* for twenty-one days. It was then to be rubbed with a little cream to make a paste. This paste was to be taken every night for six months. Pandit Dubey's patient, the recipient of this paste, was the husband of one of my maids. It was I who lent the emerald in question—and it was a happy maid who returned me that stone. So who am I to doubt the Pandit?

He told me something else about emeralds too: emeralds of quality are supposed to change color if they come in contact with poison. That is one reason, said he, that the Mughal rulers of India took their alcohol in emerald

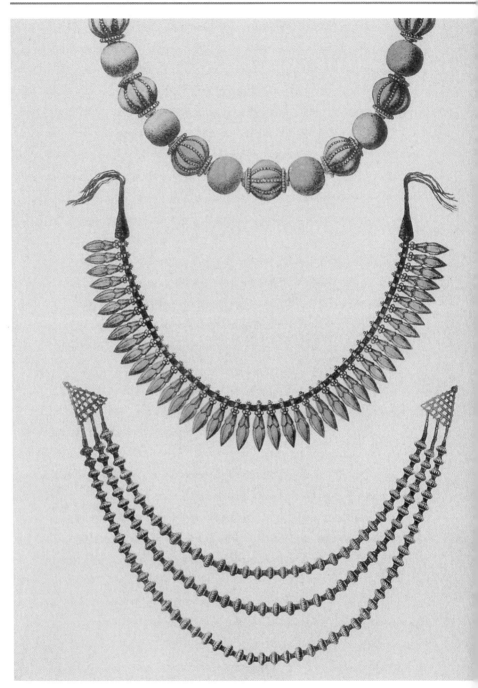

Silver, gold and jeweled necklaces and armlets

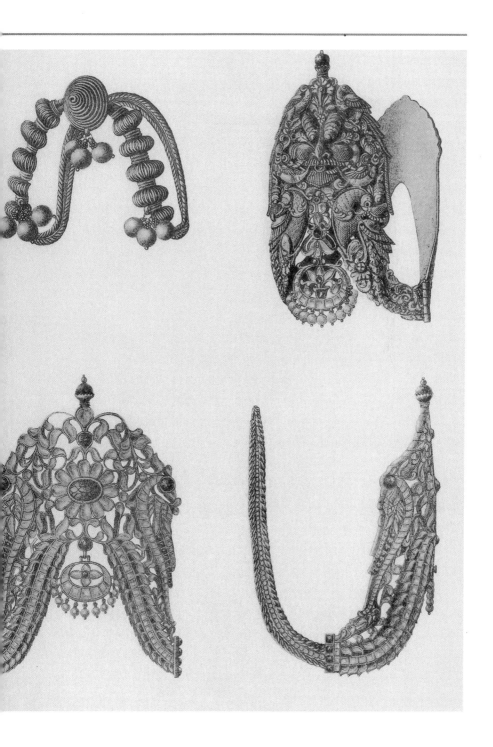

glasses. The other reason was that one can apparently drink great quantities of alcohol from emerald glasses without feeling inebriated.

It fascinates me, this so called science of stones, yet I don't know how true it is. They say diamonds have all sorts of attributes apart from stimulating the libido. Women who want a son wear them in good faith. Insomniacs believe they induce sleep. Some singers swear by diamonds to preserve their vocal cords. The list of claims goes on and on.

Almost every gemstone has some wondrous quality according to those who believe. Powdered cat's eye is said to be a cure for impotency; whole cat's eye worn next to the skin reduces blood sugar levels in diabetics! How have we worked out such things?

One woman in the Madanpur *zenana* told me a very precise remedy should I ever have bad breath: hold a topaz in my mouth for fifteen minutes in the morning before the sun rose. Another claimed that anyone could clear her complexion and overcome body odor by wearing a zircon next to her skin. Water in which a zircon had been soaked was, according to her, also very beneficial for barren women.

One gets a bit bewildered thinking about which stone affects a particular ailment. Some people try to cover all their bets by wearing a *navratna. Navratna* means simply "nine gems" that are usually cast into a pendant or ring. Those nine stones are considered by *vaids* to be particularly auspicious and beneficial. The classic setting for the *navratna* is a center ruby surrounded by pearl, topaz, coral, emerald, diamond, sapphire, zircon, and cat's eye.

Together these nine gems take care of any evil influences the planets might exert on their wearer. They give that wearer everything she desires: long life, wealth, success, prestige, family happiness, sons, and mental peace. They also, it is claimed, protect from sickness, but only on condition that the stones in the set be flawless. Second-rate stones are not strong enough to counterbalance the influence of the planets. In the olden days, jewelers graded stones into castes, just as our society graded people. People in the trade would classify a stone as priest, warrior, trader, craftsman, and menial castes, instead of saying excellent, very good, good, fair, and average.

The settings were as important as the stones. To be effective, the stones must be set so that they touch the wearer's skin at all times. The metals that hold them must be carefully chosen to suit the wearer's constitution and nature, as well as his horoscope.

I have already spoken about our belief in the beneficial qualities of metals and our consequent preference for gold necklaces, silver eating and drinking utensils, and copper vessels for storing bathing and drinking water. Pandit Dubey explained that these beliefs about the various metals are deeply ingrained in the psyche of both sexes.

As always, he quoted from his favorite *Sushruta* about the various qualities of the different metals. "Gold has a sweet and agreeable taste, acts as a tonic, imparts rotundity to the body, and subdues the action of all the three deranged humours of the body." I have already mentioned those three components: earth and water *(kapham)*, space and air *(vatam)*, and energy and water *(pittam)*. Gold is cooling in its potency and invigorates the eyesight.

About silver, *Sushruta* says, "It has an acid taste, is laxative and cooling, and destroys *pittam* and *vayu* (wind)." And so our lampblack was always kept in silver boxes, which imparted their cooling properties to eyesight. "Copper," says *Sushruta,* "has a sweet and astringent taste and acts as a liquifacient and corrosive agent, it is laxative and cooling in its potency." *Kasha*, the alloy of five metals with which the maids rubbed my feet, "has a bitter taste, is liquifacient and subdues the *kapham* and *vayu* and is beneficial to eyesight. Iron generates *vayu*, is cooling in its potency, allays thirst and subdues the deranged *pittam* and *kapham*. Zinc and lead are vermifugal as well as liquifacient and corrosive and have a saline taste."

I don't think many laymen understand all this; I must confess that I don't, but jewelers and astrologers seem to. They not only advise which stone one should wear, but also the metal in which it should be set: gold, silver, copper, steel, or brass. A mixture of all these metals is called *panchadhatu*. Many people want all five of those metals to be in contact with their

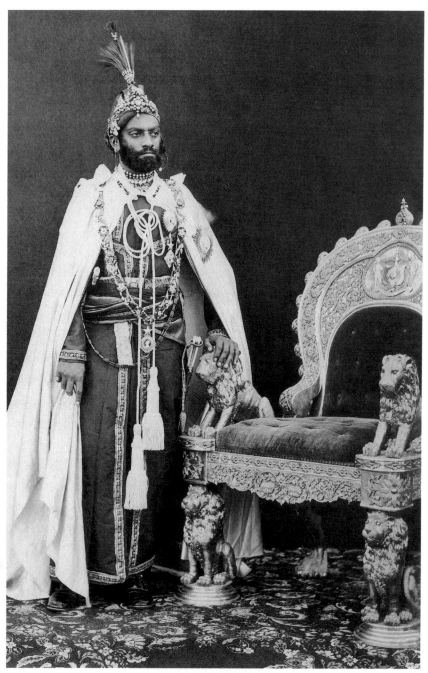

Maharana of Udaipur

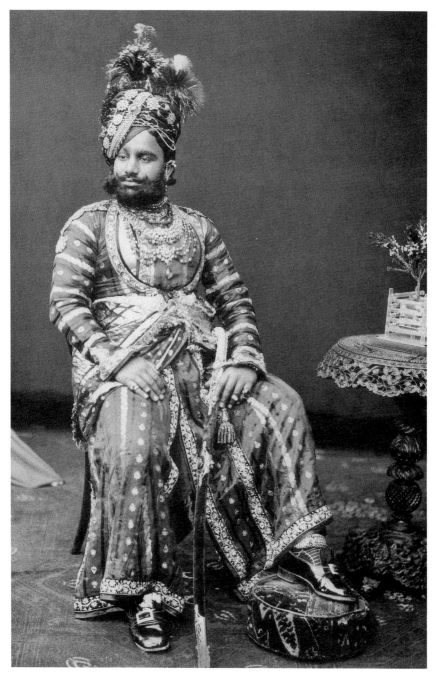

Raja of Ratlam

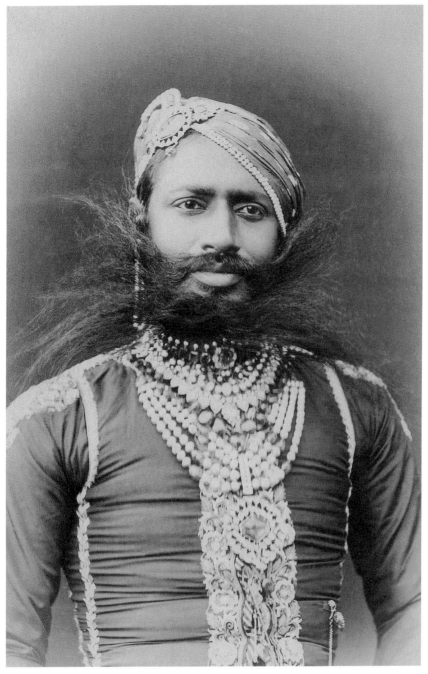

Raja of Shahpura

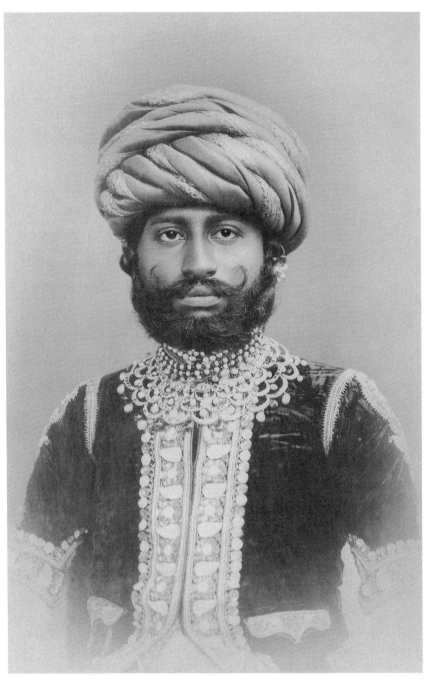

Thakur Sahib of Morvi

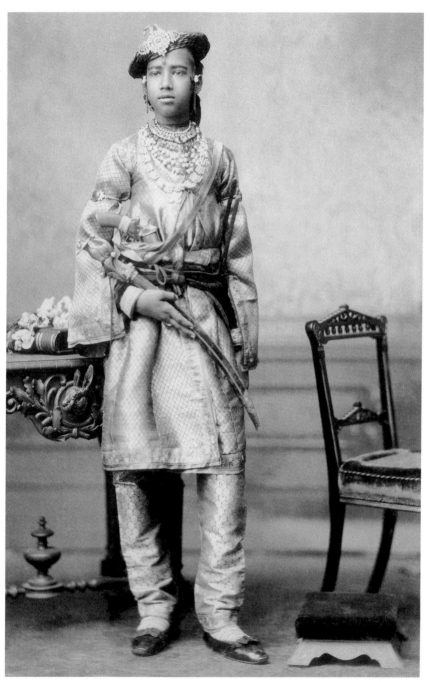

Raja of Charkhari

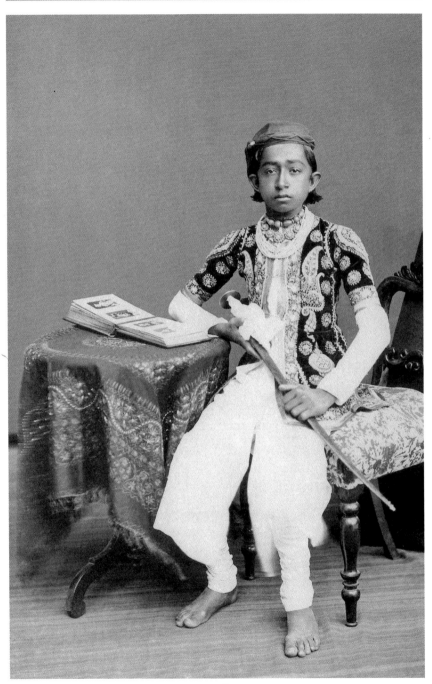

Maharana of Jhalawar

bodies so they wear them in some form of jewelry, usually a ring. Steel and brass have a higher melting point than the three other metals, so jewelers solve this problem by making the band of copper, silver, and gold and using rivets of steel and brass.

My own astrologer recommended I wear emeralds and pearls set in gold. That suited me fine, as these are my favorites. For me pearls, especially the pearls of Basra, have such beauty and such lovely memories. Pearls will always remind me of Sharad Purnima, the full moon night. Pearls and ash of pearls are said to have innumerable healing properties. Perhaps that is why many brides in the old days bathed in water in which pearls had been soaked.

his reminds me of a story. When I was a newly married bride in Madanpur, my grandfather used to come and visit me from time to time. He was a very humble man, my mother's father. As I have said, my origins are far more modest than my husband's, though my father's clan is higher than his. As a humble and a very simple man, my grandfather was free from many of the pretensions we Rajput royals used to affect. He would come to visit me in a simple bullock cart. Though I always offered to send him a car from the palace, he said he was content with his cart.

As my mother was the youngest of many children, my grandfather was quite aged by the time of my marriage. He walked with difficulty and his eyes often failed him. But he carried himself proudly and always refused when anyone offered to escort him up the stairs to my apartments in the palace.

I would come immediately whenever my maid brought word to me that he had arrived. In spite of my protests, he always rose when I entered the room. "You are a great princess now, my little one. Your father-in-law owns the throne of this state; I must pay my respects to you always." So he would fold his hands in a *namaskar* before sitting with me and taking my hand for a chat.

If he noticed that I was not wearing any anklets or if he took my hand and felt there were no bangles, he would admonish me lovingly and say, "Darling child, why are you wearing no jewelry? I have even blessed your head and there are no earrings, no necklace. That is wrong. You must always adorn yourself to welcome Lakshmi. People must live according to their status." His generation really believed that.

If I was not wearing jewelry, it was only because he had come unexpectedly, and I had just emerged from my bath. Normally I wore all the ornaments required by my status. In those days I had no desire to either hurt my beloved grandfather or to offend my own family! I wore everything expected of me. Much of it had come in my dowry as my *stree-dhan* and my mother had been careful to explain the significance of every piece that I wore.

The *tikka* pendant, which I wore on the center of my forehead with a string of pearls through my hair parting, must remind me, she said, always to walk on the straight path through life. My earrings must remind me not to have weak ears, not to listen to gossip or idle conversation (I never wore earrings in the bath!). My anklets and toe-rings were to guide me in putting the right foot forward with every step in life; my nose ring, which in those days was quite large and heavy, must bring to mind a saying of ours: "The pearl should not be heavier than the nose," that is, your spending should not outweigh your income.

My necklaces, as I have said, were to remind me that my head should stay humbly bowed, and my bangles, rich and gold on my wrists, should always be stretched forward in acts of charity. I loved my mother's favorite saying and tried to take it to heart: "Feet are made pure by pilgrimage, the hands by charity, and the lips by calling on God."

She used to be after the woman who massaged us children to concentrate on the girls' little hands, knead them so that they would be supple enough to accept the most slender of bangles. I remember the *bangriwallis*, the bangle-sellers who came to fill our wrists with the delicate glass bangles. They would squeeze the knuckles of the hands in such a manner as to put the smallest possible size of bangles onto our wrists. We Indian women admire very slender hands. We love wrists covered in bangles, but they must hug the hands so snugly as never to clang. Bangles must only jingle discreetly whenever a woman moves her hand. I never dared explain that to Miss Blake. Poor

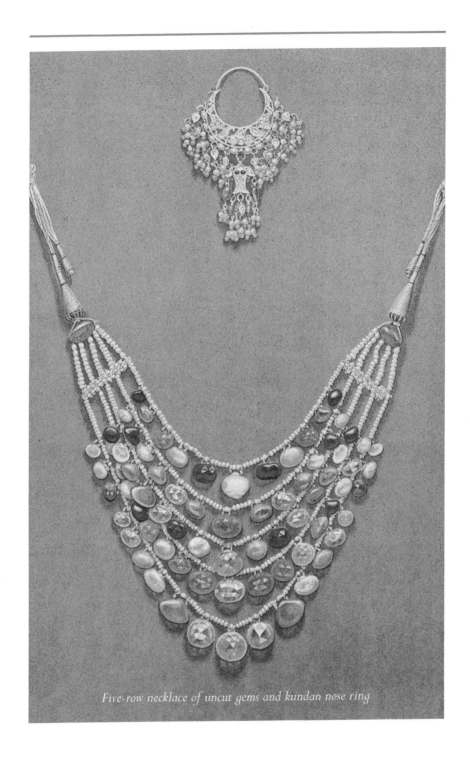

Five-row necklace of uncut gems and kundan nose ring

thing, her hands and wrists were so big, we never could find any bangles to fit her unless they were made specially, and even then, to fit over her hands, they had to be so wide that once on the wrists, they clanged about most indiscreetly.

My massage woman, Jijabai, brought Miss Blake some green glass bangles when she announced she would marry Major McBride. Green glass bangles are a tradition in Jijabai's birthplace, Maharashtra. They are supposed to represent fertility. A widow must not wear them, just as she must not wear a green *sari* or any jewelry for that matter. Miss Blake's glass bangles broke, one by one, as we tried to slip them over her hand and onto her wrist. I was always glad she never knew how inauspicious it was to break these fertility symbols, but in any case somehow she did have a child and a happy married life.

Maybe foreigners' planets are different. Or perhaps it was because Pandit Dubey prescribed such an excellent stone for her to wear; the diamond we all gave her as a wedding present. I believe she never ever took it off. Diamonds are well known, as I have said, for increasing one's potency and protecting their wearer from harm.

Aside from that stone and the small gold band Major McBride gave her, I think Miss Blake had only her big watch and pair of pearl earrings to her name. All the *zenana* women were curious about this. In our way of thinking, when a woman married, she must bring along as much jewelry as her parents could afford. Jewelry was the dowry after all. Clothes, money, and property were of much less importance to us.

There is intense curiosity in the *zenana* about what jewelry a new bride will bring. No one has any inhibitions about asking the most pointed questions about the dowry jewelry: how much was it worth? Were the stones real? Was it set by a famous jeweler? Did the gold come from family wealth or was it purchased in the market? On and on and on went the questions. Miss Blake was appalled by our lack of discretion; but among us, such knowledge was considered public property; we all felt it was our right to know.

Still, I remember experiencing acute embarrassment as a new bride in Madanpur. So many pairs of eyes were examining me, appraising the value of my jewelry, expertly estimating its worth to the last little toe-ring. No wonder my eyes were downcast. I was also very uncomfortable because custom dictates that a new bride must wear as much jewelry as can be loaded on her body. I could hardly move; I was stiff with ornaments and exhausted by their weight in addition to my heavy brocade garments.

I was wearing the heavy *timaniya* choker, a necklace that is traditionally put around a Rajasthani bride's neck by her mother. It was exquisitely crafted. On the front side, emeralds, uncut diamonds, and pearls were intricately patterned in bands of gold. On the reverse side were iridescent floral designs of enamel in green, blue, and gold, which always reminded me of the peacocks who strutted around in the palace gardens. Someone told me that it was the Mughals who introduced this type of *jadao* setting to India.

On top of all this, I was wearing *choodas*. *Choodas* are heavy bangles of ivory, worn from the wrist right up to the elbow. By tradition, they are the most important jewelry worn by a bride in Rajasthan, though they are far from the most expensive. Those ivory *choodas* are all dyed red, but for one; that one for some reason is green. The story I was told is that long ago married women wore ivory bangles to show the world that their husbands were so brave they could go out and shoot elephants!

Better that, I suppose, than the tradition in Bengal, where married women wear a bangle, not of ivory, but of plain old iron, plated with a thin wash of gold. That iron bangle is supposed to ensure the long life of their husbands. No one seems to know why. To me it seems more likely to ensure the wife's own long life, as the gold wears into her skin over the years, imparting its beneficial qualities. In any case, she must remove the

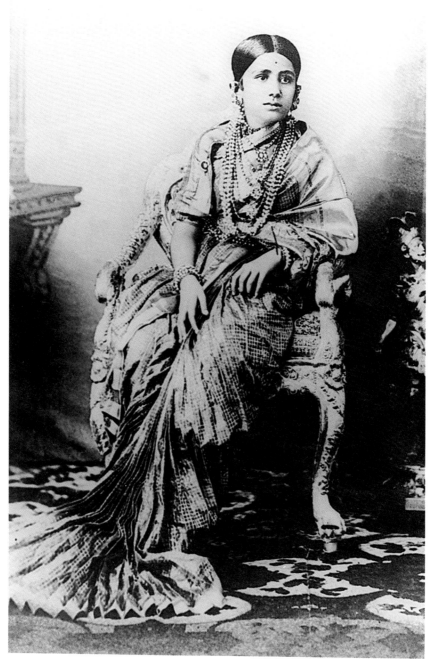

Maharani of Mysore

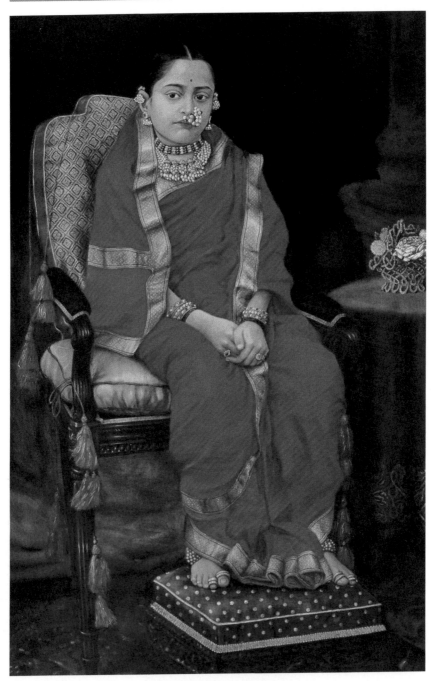

Princess Tarabai of Baroda

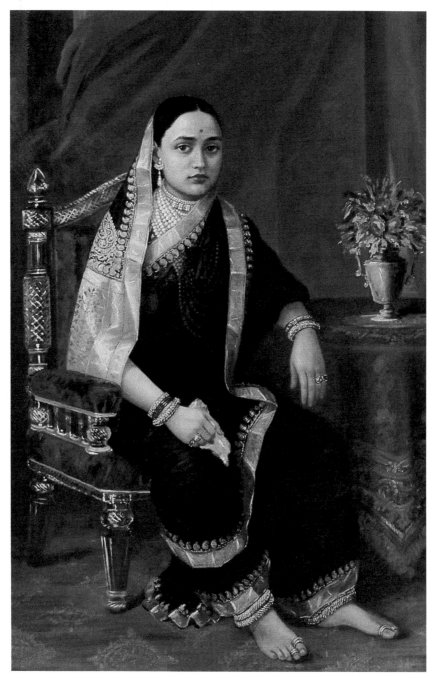

Maharani Chimanbai II of Baroda

bangle if she becomes a widow. Similarly, most Indian women must, by custom, remove their jewelry when their husbands depart for the next world.

We do not have wedding rings. Many Hindu women wear a necklace called *mangalsutra* to show they are married. *Mangal* means auspicious and *sutra* means thread. Today *mangalsutras* are made from all sorts of things including precious stones, but originally they were made of simple thread dyed in saffron, tied into three knots and strung with tiny black beads. Each area of India and each community has its own variation of the *mangalsutra*. In the South Indian state of Kerala, for example, a *mangalsutra* is called a *tali*. It is made of 108 strands of gold wire, woven together and washed with saffron before it is tied on the bride. Kashmiri brides wear their wedding rings in their ears. The *dajehroo*, which is bejeweled and heavy, dangles from the earlobes; the *atehroo* is a long thread of silver or gold that is wound around the ear to support the weight of the *dajehroo*.

Married women in many regions must also wear silver toe-rings. They are worn on the second and third toes of each foot because we believe that the nerves of these two particular toes connect with the reproductive organs and therefore make a woman more fertile. Miss Blake claimed this at least made more sense than the green glass bangles because toes are in fact connected to nerves that branch to the reproductive organs, just as nerves in the western ring finger are directly connected to the heart.

In addition to toe-rings, married women of my mother's generation wore so many different earrings all at one time that they almost covered the whole outer ear from the top to the lobe. In Rajasthan, each type of earring on various parts of the ear has a different name. I have never worn all of them, but I am familiar with the names: *jhabrak, kundal,* and *patta.*

Each one was worn at a specific point on the ear. There were those who believed that each of these points was important and putting the correct metal through each could prevent such sufferings as migraine, sinusitis, and certain allergies. Some even claimed that piercing the ears or the nose in particular places could temper the nature of a difficult woman and render her more docile!

I don't know about that or, for that matter, about any of these so-called theories. But I do know that Indians have loved jewelry since their earliest history. Look at our sculptures, frescoes, and paintings; men and women alike are covered in jewelry—not just one piece, but as much as their bodies could support. Whereas Miss Blake found it ostentatious and vulgar, we found anything that was not heavily adorned to be ugly and inauspicious.

By the time I came to Madanpur, it was considered impractical to wear mountains of jewelry during the day, like some of those ancient sculptures. It was also faintly suggestive of the women who danced at our durbars—not really courtesans, but not women of virtue.

That did not mean we looked down on jewelry—far from it. On festival days we were issued as much jewelry as we desired. Miss Blake was absolutely astonished the first time she went with me to visit the *toshakhana*. The *toshakhana* was the treasury where all state property like jewelry was kept. Everything was listed in yard-long notebooks, each issue recorded meticulously. Usually it was the senior Maharani who dictated who was to wear which set of jewelry for important occasions when we all dressed up.

In the company of a very old aunt, Miss Blake and I were once shown box after box of pearls the size of marbles, rubies like pigeon's blood, emeralds and diamonds the size of a thumbnails, and sapphires blue like the sea. The keeper opened these boxes one after the other. Then he opened a big velvet-lined case that I had not seen before.

That ancient auntie smiled a very tiny smile and raised up its lid. With old hands and a little girl's smile, she lifted its contents and put them on me; a full garment of gold chains: yards and yards of them intricately linked. I was literally covered in gold: my arms, my chest, right down to my thighs. Auntie said, "This belonged to a beautiful woman much beloved of His Highness' grandfather, though her calling was the oldest in the world."

"Auntie, this is lovely!" I said. I really meant that; it was like wearing a web of spun gold. "But dear aunt, it's rather inconvenient, if you know

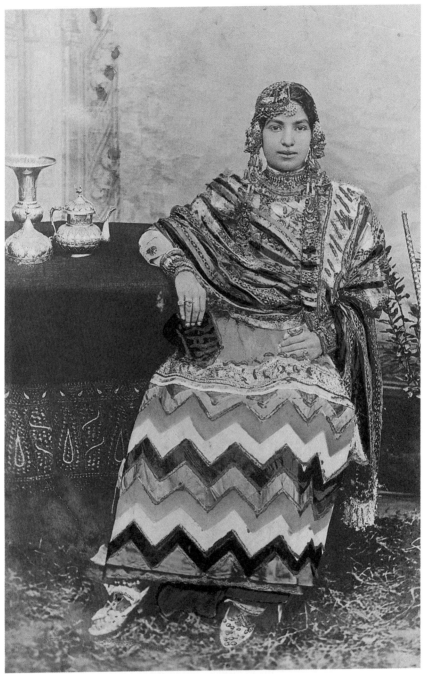

Courtesan in all her finery

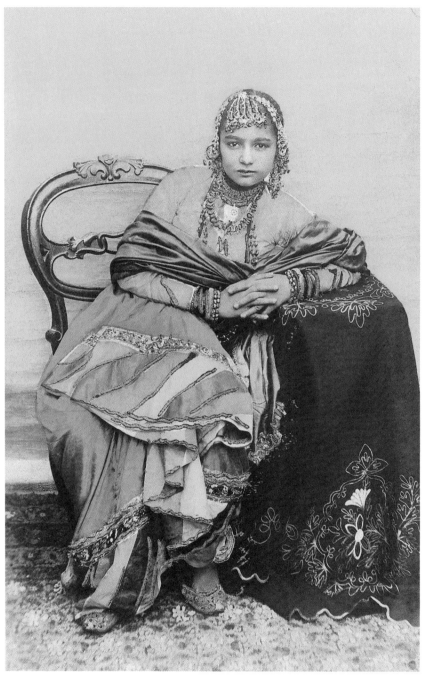

Heavily decked courtesan

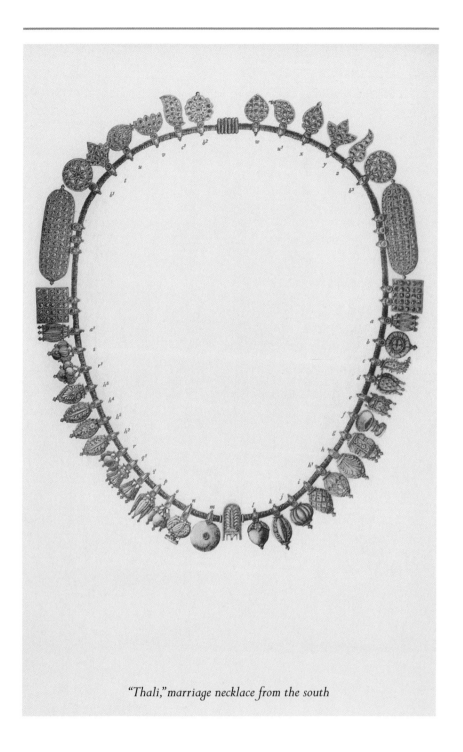

"Thali," marriage necklace from the south

what I mean. It must take hours to extricate oneself; you couldn't be in a hurry!"

Without a word, my aunt covered her head with her *sari*, stood very straight, and touched a tiny clasp near my throat. The entire piece dropped away from my shoulders and slipped to the ground, shimmering.

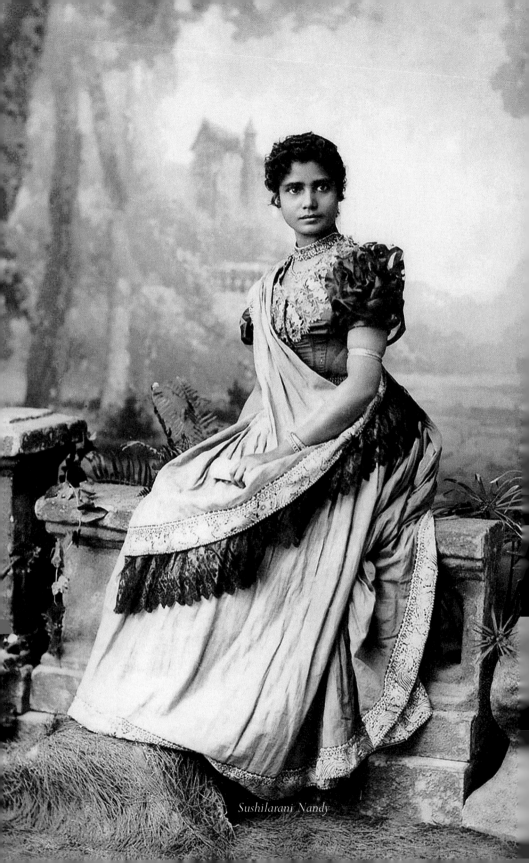

Sushilarani Nandy

11.

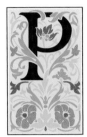

Precious Memories

Perhaps all my memories are like that necklace: fragile and beautiful and far too precious to ever be of much use today. I must put them away, back in their chest, but somehow I just don't want to end. This book has become my friend, like all my other rituals. So I must remind myself that its end is its beginning because someone may take my advice. Even those who don't will have the knowledge in their hearts: knowing is half the pleasure, and knowing means these ideas will live, even if it's just in our hearts.

I will close with one last memory, the memory of a *puja* we used to perform in the name of *roop* or beauty. Our *puja* took place fifteen days after Sharad Purnima on Roop Chaudus day, the special day when we rolled wicks for our *kaajal* from full-moon cotton. We women rose before dawn, bathed with our favorite oils and *utanas*. A bit of auspicious full-moon water was added to the water we bathed in and the jewelry that we wore had been purchased on the day of Dhanteras, the day before Roop Chaudus. Dhanteras is the most favorable day of the year for buying new jewelry. The next day was devoted to the celebration of beauty in all its aspects.

We thrived on such sweet reminders. Even if throughout the rest of the year we hadn't time to think of ourselves for one moment, on that day we were all beautiful. I know they say, "You can't quench your thirst by licking dewdrops," but the freshness of a dewdrop, one special day in the year, stayed in our hearts for many months after.

I think of this little book as an auspicious drop—a sort of printed *puja* for anyone to pick up and celebrate a moment with me.

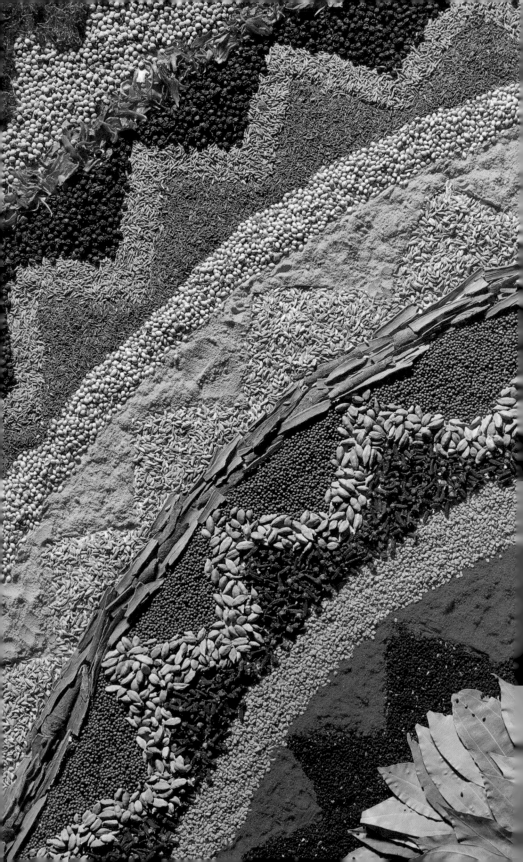

12.

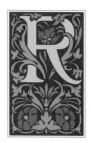ecipes

I mentioned in the introduction that I do not know if the treatments and recipes I have collected over the years always work. But trying them could be fun on a rainy or dull day or a holiday. Why not pamper yourself?

Many recipes are time-tested, but do remember that we should all be careful about allergies to certain products—sometimes even natural ones. I have written these recipes exactly as my friends and family members recounted them or jotted them down. There is no organized presentation and I know my granddaughter would not approve. But do remember, they're good for you—or so I think!

THE FACE

Do not apply any of the following face packs in the delicate area around the eyes.

SANDALWOOD For all types of skins: Grind together 1 teaspoon each of poppy seeds, *khuskhus,* and sandalwood powder with 3 almonds. Apply the paste on the face and leave for 20 minutes. Wash off with lukewarm water. To make larger quantities, use the three ingredients in equal proportions. Pound and powder, mix together and bottle. To make the pack, take 2 to 3 teaspoons of the powder and mix into a thick paste with sufficient milk. Poppy seeds and almonds are rich in oils and nutrients while sandalwood is cooling.

HONEY & EGG For oily skin: beat together until creamy, 1 tablespoon of honey with the white of 1 egg. Apply to the face and wash off with cold water after half an hour.

For dry or normal skin: beat only the yolk with honey. Wash with cold water after half an hour.

CHICKPEA FLOUR* For dry skin: Mix 1 teaspoon chickpea or moong flour, ¼ teaspoon turmeric powder, 1 teaspoon cold milk or cream. Apply on the face and neck and let dry. Wet fingertips with cold water and gently rub off, then wash with water. The pack stimulates the skin and leaves it soft and smooth. For oily skin: use water or lemon juice instead of milk to mix the pack. *Some skins may be allergic to chickpea flour. Substitute with husked green gram (moong) flour.

ALMOND-SAFFRON For cleaning skin: Rub 2 or 3 almonds on a marble slab or a *sahan* with plain water or rose water. Powder a couple of strands of saffron or dissolve them in a few drops of warm water and add to the almond paste. Apply the paste to the face and let it dry. Wet hands with water and rub the face until all the paste comes off. All dirt and dead skin will come off with the paste.

MASOOR (Whole black lentils) To remove freckles and keep skin clear of blemishes: Soak 1 teaspoon of *masoor* in 1 teaspoon of water for half an hour. Grind together with 1 teaspoon of clarified butter and apply on face. Follow this treatment for seven days.

MULTANI MITTI For smooth skin: Take a small lump of *multani mitti* (Fuller's earth, available at most Indian grocers) and dissolve in sufficient water to make a smooth paste. Apply the paste on face and neck, but not in the area around the eyes. Lie down and relax with thin slices of cucumber or cotton wool swabs soaked in rose water on the eyes. Avoid talking or smiling until the clay dries and hardens. Wash off gently with water.

MULTANI MITTI-CUCUMBER For oily skin: Thoroughly mix together 2 table-spoons each, cucumber juice, milk, and *multani mitti*. Apply on face and wash off when dry.

MANJISHTHA (Madder root) For curing acne and for soothing burns: Rub a piece of *manjishtha* root on a rubbing stone with 1 teaspoon of clarified butter. Apply to face.

PAPAYA For oily skin: Mash 1 or 2 teaspoons of ripe papaya fruit and apply on the face. Lie down for 15 minutes, then wash with water. Papain, the enzyme present in the fruit, helps remove dry and dead cells on the skin.

PAPAYA-MINT-TEA For acne and pimples: Mix one portion pulp of ripe or unripe papaya, half portion of mint leaves, and a few tea leaves. Boil all the ingredients together with three times the quantity of water. Gently dab the liquid on affected spots using either a soft piece of cloth or a cotton swab. Let dry and then wash with lukewarm water.

CREAM & HONEY For dry skin and wrinkles: Mix together 1 teaspoon each of cream and honey and massage the mixture into the face and neck. Wash with warm water after 15 minutes.

OATMEAL & HONEY For removing summer tan or dark circles around the eyes: beat together equal proportions of oatmeal, honey, white of egg, and almond oil and thoroughly massage into the face and neck, arms and legs. Wash off the pack after 20 minutes.

LEMON JUICE & HONEY For oily and lifeless skin: Mix together 1 teaspoon of lemon juice with 2 teaspoons of honey. Apply to the face and neck and wash off after 15 minutes. The pack stimulates and refreshes the skin.

BETEL LEAF For removing warts on the body or face: Do not use near the eyes. Remove the stem of a betel leaf and force out a drop of juice from the cut end with the aid of tweezers or with the fingertips. Gently touch the stem to *chunam* (slaked lime used in *paan*) and apply on the wart. Leave for about half an hour and then wash off. Apply twice a day for three or four days until the wart falls off. If there is even a slight burning sensation on application, use only once a day.

POST-NATAL

For any woman, the months after childbirth are extremely important. That is when women of my generation focused on getting their own bodies healthy and also ensuring they had sufficient milk for their little ones.

SOOJI KA HALWA: This strength-imparting delicious sweet is given to the new mother on the tenth day after childbirth. Ingredients: 2 cups semolina (*sooji* or *rawa*), 1¾ cups sugar, ½ cup *ghee* (clarified butter), a few strands of saffron, 4 cardamoms, powdered (optional), a few chopped almonds and sultanas. Lightly brown the semolina in the ghee in a heavy *kadhai* or wok. Keep stirring until thoroughly roasted. Add sufficient water to cover semolina. When it begins to steam, mix in sugar, stirring all the while. When steam rises again, pound saffron threads in a pestle and mortar and add to pan. Add cardamom, almonds, and sultanas. Stir and cook until all the water dries up.

SOOJI KI KHEER: Mix thoroughly 1 cup semolina in 1 cup of milk. Add 1 teaspoon of sugar and cook over low heat until slightly thick.

CRESS OR AHLIV KHEER: Over low heat, mix together 1 cup each of whole milk and thick coconut milk. When it begins to boil, add 2 tablespoons each cress seeds and sugar or jaggery (*gur*) and stir until thick. *Ahliv* seeds strengthen the back and enhances lactation.

CRESS & ROSE WATER: Soak 1 teaspoon cress seeds in a little rose water. Refrigerate overnight. Add to 1 cup milk with sugar to taste.

AHLIV LADDOOS (Sweet Cress Balls) Ingredients: 2 fresh coconuts, ¾ cup *ahliv* (cress) seeds, 2½ cups sugar or jaggery. Soak cress seeds in 1 cup of fresh coconut water or in ¾ cup of whole milk for 2 hours. Grate coconuts and mix with the seeds and sugar. Heat the mixture over a low heat in a heavy skillet or wok until all the liquid evaporates. When cool shape into small balls, about 2 inches in diameter.

METHI LADDOOS (Fenugreek Balls) Ingredients: ¾ cup powdered fenugreek seeds, ½ cup *ghee* (clarified butter), 1½ cups whole grain or gram flour (*atta*), ¾ cup poppy seeds, 2½ cups dried, desiccated coconut, 10 almonds chopped fine, 5 cups sugar or jaggery. Soak powdered fenugreek seeds in heated clarified butter and leave for 3 days. Roast flour in a little clarified butter and thoroughly mix in all ingredients. Knead the mixture and form into small balls. Since fenugreek is bitter, the quantity of sugar or jaggery may be increased if necessary to 6 cups. Though bitter, these *laddoos* are strength-giving and help in emptying the uterus after childbirth.

METHI BHAJI 1 (Cooked fenugreek greens) Ingredients: 3 teaspoons cooking oil, 1 bunch *methi* leaves plucked from the stem and thoroughly washed in a colander, ¼ cup washed moong *daal* (husked green gram), sugar and salt to taste. Heat the oil in a frying pan or wok and add *methi* leaves. Fry thoroughly and add 1½ cups water. Bring to a boil and add moong *daal*. When the *daal* is almost cooked, add sugar and salt to taste.

METHI BHAJI 2 (Cooked fenugreek greens) Ingredients: 2 bunches *methi* leaves, plucked from the stem and thoroughly washed, 1 teaspoon salt, 2 onions, 2 green chilies (optional), 6 cloves garlic, 2 tablespoons oil, 1 tablespoon dried desiccated coconut. Place plucked *methi* leaves in a bowl and sprinkle with salt. Rub in the salt by crushing the leaves and let stand for 15 minutes. Wash the leaves in a colander and squeeze out the water. Separately chop fine the onions, chilies, and garlic. Heat the oil in a frying pan or wok. Add chopped garlic and fry lightly until light gold in color. Add chopped onions and fry until brown and crisp. Add *methi* leaves, coconut, chopped chilies, and salt to taste. Fry until the *methi* leaves exude their aroma.

GOND OR DINK LADDOOS (Gum Arabic) Ingredients: ½ pound gum arabic, 1 pound dried desiccated coconut, ¾ cup poppy seeds, 10 almonds, 1 pound dried fruit (pistachios, cashew nuts, dates, walnuts, sultanas, raisins, etc.), ½ cup *ghee* or clarified butter, 4–5 cups sugar. Coarsely pound the gum arabic. Roast the coconut and poppy seeds separately on a lightly greased griddle or tawa. Skin the almonds by soaking in a little water, and chop finely. Chop dried fruit. Deep-fry the gum arabic in clarified butter until it puffs up. Drain off excess butter. Heat sugar and 1 cup water to make syrup and then add clarified butter. Add all other ingredients and form into small balls while hot. Gum arabic strengthens the bones.

GINGER SOUP: Heat to smoking point 1 teaspoon of *ghee* or any cooking oil in a small skillet or frying pan. Add a small pinch of powdered asafoetida (*hing*) and ½ teaspoon each of dried ginger powder (*sonth*) and cumin seed. When the seeds sputter, add to 1 cup of warm milk and stir. This delicious soup prevents colds in the breast-feeding mother.

MEAT SOUP Ingredients: ½ cup moong *daal* (husked green gram), 1 cup rice, ½ pound finely minced mutton or beef, 1 bunch each spinach (*palak*) and dill (*suwa*) leaves, washed and chopped, 1 large onion, 4 cloves garlic, 2 tablespoons cooking oil, salt to taste. Thoroughly wash and soak moong *daal* and rice in a skillet with water to cover by 1 inch. Leave for 30 minutes. Add meat and greens and cook over low heat until meat is tender. Stir thoroughly. Skin and chop fine onion and garlic. In a small frying pan, heat the oil and add onions and fry until golden brown. Remove from heat and add to the soup. Salt to taste. The soup is very nourishing for mothers who are breastfeeding their babies.

ATTA LADDOOS (Whole wheat flour) Ingredients: ½ cup + 2 tablespoons *ghee* (clarified butter), 5 cups whole-wheat flour, 7 ounces gum arabic (*gond, dink*), ½ cup dried, grated (or desiccated) coconut, ½ cup poppy seeds, (khuskhus), 2½ cups castor sugar. Heat 2 tablespoons of clarified butter in a skillet and roast flour until golden. Heat the remaining ½ cup clarified butter and fry gum arabic until puffed and pound into a fine powder. Roast coconut and poppy seeds on a griddle until light brown. Mix and knead together all ingredients and shape into 1-inch balls. These *laddoos* are very nourishing and also aid lactation.

AMBOLI (Rice pancakes) Ingredients: 1 cup rice flour, ½ teaspoon powdered fenugreek seeds, ¼ teaspoon salt, ¼ teaspoon baking powder. Place all ingredients in a deep pan and add enough water to make a paste of pouring consistency, but not too thin. Cover and keep for about 3 hours to let the dough rise. Heat 1 tablespoon of oil in a heavy griddle or *tawa* or use a non-stick frying pan. Pour in about 3 tablespoons of the mixture. Cover with a lid and let cook until a weblike pattern forms on the surface. Alternatively, instead of using rice flour and powdered seeds, soak the rice and fenugreek seeds overnight in a little water, and grind to a paste the next morning. Serve with a pat of butter as a tea-time snack. *Ambolis* aid lactation.

BREWS & TONICS
Useful for a variety of ailments and for general well-being, these decoctions are most effective when freshly made.

MIXED SPICES: For loss of appetite, powder equal quantities of cinnamon, dried ginger (*sonth*), and cardomoms (*elaichi*), sieve through muslin. Take ½ teaspoon of the powder mixed with honey, before meals.

GULKAND: Remove petals from sufficient quantity of fragrant pink roses— the wild variety is excellent. Place ¼ inch deep layer of petals in a large, glass jar. Top with a layer of rock candy (*khadisakhar* or *misri*). Continue to alternate layers of petals and rock candy until the jar is full. Tightly close the lid and place in the sun or in a warm place for 15 days. Then let stand for 2 months before opening the jar. Take 1 teaspoon morning and evening. *Gulkand* is especially given to young children to prevent constipation.

Because of its cooling properties, it makes an ideal food supplement after fevers or sunstroke.

EIGHT POWDERS (*Ashtachoorna*): Roast equal quantities of dried ginger (*sonth*), asafoetida (*hing*), black pepper, long pepper, celery seed, black cumin seeds (*shahzeera*), cumin seeds, and rock salt on a heavy iron griddle or *tawa*. Remove from heat and let cool. Pound into a powder and sieve. Put the *ashtachoorna* in a tightly lidded jar. Add ¼ teaspoon of the powder to a glass of salted buttermilk or to the juice of half a sour lime. It's good for indigestion, acidity, and coughs.

SARSAPARILLA DECOCTION (*Anantmool kadha*): Mash 2 tablespoons of *anatmool* or *upalsari* root (sarsaparilla) in 4 cups of water. Boil until reduced to ½ cup. Add sugar or rock candy. This is a good remedy for waning appetite, urinary disorders, itches, and skin allergies.

PANCHAMRIT Ingredients: 2 parts lime or lemon juice, 1½ parts fresh ginger juice, 1 part juice of fresh mint leaves, 1½ parts rock candy (*misri*), 1 part rock salt, ½ part powdered asafoetida (*hing*). Mix all the ingredients together and cook over low heat until the mixture thickens. Strain, cool, and bottle. Take 1 teaspoonful for acidity and indigestion or for restoring appetite after a long illness.

ADRAK PAK (Ginger fudge): Wash, peel, and cut into pieces ½ pound fresh ginger and then grind to a fine consistency. Stir in 2½ times the quantity of sugar (about 3½ cups). Place the mixture in a heavy pan and cook over a low heat, stirring constantly. When the edges of the pan begin to turn white, remove from heat. Mix in 2 teaspoons castor sugar and 2 teaspoons lime juice (optional). Lightly grease a flat pan and pat the mixture evenly into ¼-inch thickness. Cut into 1-inch squares. When cool, remove squares and bottle. It's effective for acidity, indigestion, morning sickness, and coughs.

TULSI KADHA 1 (Basil tea): Add to 2 cups of water: 10 basil leaves, 2–3 tender blossoms of basil (optional), 3 cloves, 2 peeled cardamoms, ¼ inch piece of fresh ginger root, 1 bael leaf (optional). Boil until reduced to ⅛ quantity. Take 2 teaspoons of warm tea at a time, several times a day, as a remedy for coughs or morning sickness.

TULSI KADHA 2 (Basil tea): 10-12 basil leaves, 2 teaspoons coriander seeds, 1 teaspoon *saunf* (anise), 2-inch piece *mulatthi* or *jeshtimadh* (Indian licorice), rock candy or sugar to taste. Boil the ingredients in 2 cups of water and reduce to ⅛ quantity.

GARLIC TONIC: Soak ½ pound garlic onions in 2 pounds natural yogurt for 24 hours. Remove and peel each pod. Fry the pods in ½ cup *ghee* (clarified butter) until they turn golden. Cool and bottle. This preparation is a good tonic to aid mending bones after a fracture and also as a remedy for laryngitis, night-blindness, or for indigestion. Dose for adults: depending on body weight, 3 to 5 pods every morning and 2 to 4 every evening. Younger children who are on solid foods are to be given ½ a pod morning and evening.

SANDALWOOD SHERBET: Soak in a large pan 2 pounds of sandalwood powder or fine shavings in good quality, fragrant rose water for 24 hours. Place the pan over low heat and remove from heat as soon as it begins to boil. Strain and add 2 pounds rock candy or sugar syrup. Cool and bottle. Take 2 teaspoons of the sherbet morning and evening. Works wonders as a strength-imparting tonic for pregnant women and undernourished children. A cooling drink in summer.

CHIRAITA KADHA (Chiretta tonic): Pound together 4 teaspoons chiretta with ¼ teaspoon of dried ginger (*sonth*). Add to 2 cups of water and boil until reduced to ⅛ quantity. Give morning and evening for high fevers, especially malaria.

GENERAL RECIPES AND INFORMATION

These are tips and suggestions on different aspects of beauty and health.

KAMAL (Lotus): Lotus flowers are blue, white, or deep pink. The lotus is a popular remedy for heart ailments. ½ teaspoon of dried and powdered flowers are mixed with an equal quantity of honey, 1 teaspoon butter, and sugar candy. A decoction of dried blue lotus petals and water is used for low-grade fever and bilious attacks.

MANJISHTHA (Madder): During the excavations at the Indus Valley, a civilization that dates back to around 3000 BC, fragments of cloth dyed in madder (*manjishtha*) were found. Besides being a popular traditional dye, the root of Indian madder is also used in beauty care in the treatment of acne and pimples and to soothe burns. Rub the root with a little clarified butter on a *sahan* or marble pastry board and apply the paste to the affected skin.

SINDUR: To make genuine *sindur* soak sticks of turmeric overnight and scrape off skin with a sharp knife. Grind together 2 teaspoons each *papadkhar* and drumsticks (*savagi*), finely sieve and mix with lemon juice. Apply to turmeric sticks which turn red. Grind sticks to *sindur* powder.

FRAGRANT SACHETS

Most of these ingredients will be available with your local pansari *or grocer. Some, like musk, are expensive and are optional. Stitch little sachets with thin, attractive pieces of cloth and fill with any one of the following:*

Sandalwood powder or sandalwood shavings; Indian patchouli (*Pogostomon pachouli*) commonly known as *panchpanadi*; vetiver grass or *khus*; spikenard, known in India as *jatamansi*.

If you wish to make a large quantity of sachets, use the following proportions for an unusual combination of a variety of fragrant herbs and spices:

Arrowroot powder 100 parts, powdered cloves 20 parts, dried and powdered orange leaves 15 parts, powdered cinnamon 10 parts, lemon oil 1 part, orange oil 1 part, ambergris ¼ part. Sieve and mix together powdered clove, cinnamon, and orange leaves; add arrowroot and ambergris, then sprinkle the oils. Mix thoroughly and fill sachets.

HERBAL FRAGRANCE: *Jatamansi* 15 parts, nagarmotha (sedge) 10 parts, *khus* grass (vetiver) 10 parts, *ood* or *agar* (eaglewood) 2 parts, camphor 1 part, musk crystal ¼ part. Pound and sieve together *jatamansi, nagarmotha, khus,* and *ood.* Add camphor powder and musk and fill sachets.

DAMP IN CUPBOARDS: Place a little *chunam* (slaked lime) in a small box on shelf.

PHOTOGRAPH CREDITS

Glossary

PLANTS, FLOWERS, SPICES, AND GRAINS

English	Indian	Latin
Almond	Badam	Prunus amygdalus
Amla	Amla/Aonla	Phyllanthus embelica
Anise	Saunf	Pimpinella anisum
Areca Nut	Supari	Areca catechu
Bael	Bel	Aegle marmelos
Banana Plantain	Kela	Musa paradisiaca
Banyan	Vad/Baad	Ficus begalensis
Barberry	Daru-halad	Berberis aristata
Basil holy or sacred	Tulsi	Ocimum sanctum
Betel leaf	Paan	Piper betle
Bishop's weed	Ajwain/Owa	Carum copticum
Bitter gourd	Karela	Momordica charantia
Black Pepper	Kali mirch	Piper nigrum
Camphor	Kapoor Karpur	Cinnamomum camphora

English	Indian	Latin
Caraway	Shahzeera	Carum carui
Cardamom	Elaichi/Velchi	Elettaria cardamomum
Cashew	Caju	Anacardium occidentale
Castor Erand	Rendi	Ricinus communis
Chebulic Myrobalan	Harda/Harad	Terminalia chebula
Chickpea	Chana	Cicer aricentinum
Cinnamon	Dalchini	Cinnamomum zeylanicum
Cloves	Lawang	Caryophyllus floribunda
Coconut	Nariyal	Cocos nucifera
Common cress seeds	Ahliv	Lepidium sativum
Coriander	Dhaniya	Coriandrum sativum
Cumin seeds	Zeera/Jeera	Cuminum cyminum
Date	Khajur	Phoenix dactyliefra
Dill greens	Suwa/Shepu	Peucedanum graveolens
Dill seeds	Balant shepa	Peucedanum graveolens
Drumstick	Shevga/Sahajan	Moringa oleifera
Eaglewood	Oodh/Loban	Styrax benzoin
Emblic Myrobalan	Amla/ Aonla	Emblica officinalis
Fenugreek	Methi	Trigonella fœnum-grœcum
Fig (sacred)	Peepal	Ficus religiosa
Frankincense	Ood/Dhup Loban	

English	Indian	Latin
Garlic	Lasan/Lehsun	Allium sativum
Ginger (fresh)	Adrak	Zingiber officinale
Ginger (dried)	Sonth/Sunth	Zingiber officinale
Grass	Harialee/Dub Durva	Cynodon dactylon
Henna	Mehndi	Lawsonia inermis
Hibiscus	Jaswand Gurhal	Hibiscus rosasinensis
Indian Madder	Manjishtha/ Manjith	Rubia cordifolia
Indian Pennywort	Brahmi	Centella asiatica
Jasmine	Mogra/Motia Chameli/Juhi	Jasminum grandiflorum
Lemongrass	Hari chai	Andropogon citratus
Lentils-black	Udad	Phaseolus radiata
Lentils-brown	Masoor	Cicer aricentium
Licorice	Mulatthi/ Jeshtimadh	Glycyrrhiza glabra
Lime	Nimbu/ Limboo	Citrus medica
Lotus	Kamal	Nelumbo nucifera
Mango	Aam/Amba	Mangifera Indica
Mango-ginger	Ambia haldi/ Am haldi	Curcuma amada
Mangosteen	Kokam/ Amsool	Garcinia indica
Margosa	Neem/Nimb	Azadirachta indica

English	Indian	Latin
Marking nut	Bibba	Semecarpus anacardium
Millet	Bajra/Jowar	Penicellaria spicata
Mung	Moong	Phaseolus mungo
Mustard	Rai/Mohori	Brassia nigra
Myrobalan	Hirada/Harada	Terminalia chebula
Myrobalan	Behda/Baheda	Terminalia bellerica
Nutmeg	Jaiphal	Myristica fragrans
Patchouli	Panch Panadi	Pogostomon pachouli
Rose	Gulab	Rosa centifolia
English	Indian	Latin
Saffron	Keshar/Kesar	Crocus sativus
Sandalwood	Chandan	Santalum album
Sandalwood Red	Lalchandan/Raktachandan	Pterocarpus santalinus
Sarsapailla	Anantmool	Hemidesmus indicus
Screwpine (fragrant)	Kevra/Keoda	Pandanus odoratissimus
Sedge	Nagarmotha	Cyperus scariosus
Soapnut	Ritha	Sapindus trifoliatus
Soapnut	Shikakai	Acacia concinna
Spikenard	Jatamansi	Nardostachys jatamansi
Spinach	Palak	Spinacea oleracea
Sweetflag	Vekhand	Acorus calamus
Tamarind	Imli/Chincha	Tamarindus indica
Turmeric	Haldi	Curcuma longa
Vetiver	Khus/Vala	Vetiveria zizanioides

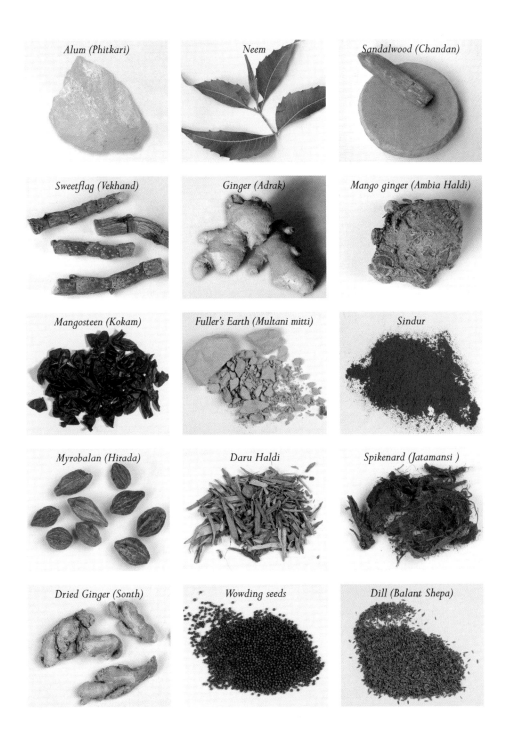

Alum (Phitkari)

Neem

Sandalwood (Chandan)

Sweetflag (Vekhand)

Ginger (Adrak)

Mango ginger (Ambia Haldi)

Mangosteen (Kokam)

Fuller's Earth (Multani mitti)

Sindur

Myrobalan (Hirada)

Daru Haldi

Spikenard (Jatamansi)

Dried Ginger (Sonth)

Wowding seeds

Dill (Balant Shepa)

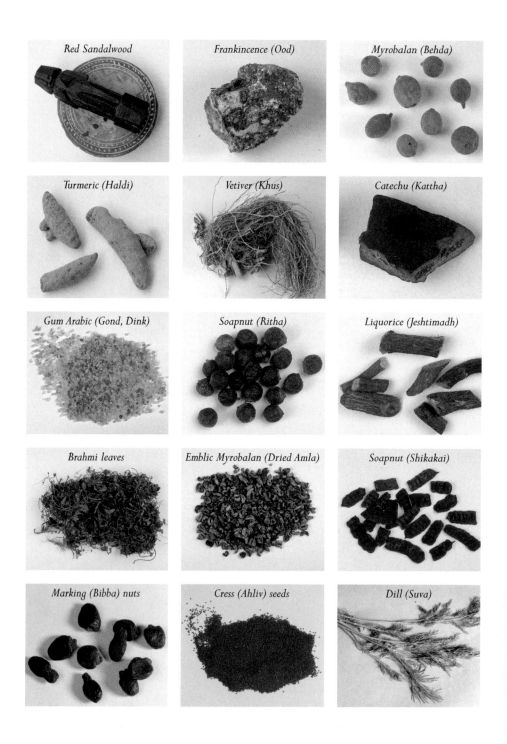

Red Sandalwood

Frankincense (Ood)

Myrobalan (Behda)

Turmeric (Haldi)

Vetiver (Khus)

Catechu (Kattha)

Gum Arabic (Gond, Dink)

Soapnut (Ritha)

Liquorice (Jeshtimadh)

Brahmi leaves

Emblic Myrobalan (Dried Amla)

Soapnut (Shikakai)

Marking (Bibba) nuts

Cress (Ahliv) seeds

Dill (Suva)